RAPID WE

MW00510503

HYPNOSIS

HOW TO LOSE WEIGHT NATURALLY, RAPIDLY, EFFORTLESSLY. THE ULTIMATE GUIDE TO CALORIES BLAST AND FAT BURN WITH SELF-HYPNOSIS AND MEDITATION, HYPNOTIC GASTRIC BAND INCLUDED.

GENA LANTZ

© Copyright 2020 - All rights reserved.

The content contained within this book may not be reproduced, duplicated or transmitted without direct written permission from the author or the publisher.

Under no circumstances will any blame or legal responsibility be held against the publisher, or author, for any damages, reparation, or monetary loss due to the information contained within this book. Either directly or indirectly.

Legal Notice:

This book is copyright protected. This book is only for personal use. You cannot amend, distribute, sell, use, quote or paraphrase any part, or the content within this book, without the consent of the author or publisher.

Disclaimer Notice:

Please note the information contained within this document is for educational and entertainment purposes only. All effort has been executed to present accurate, up to date, and reliable, complete information. No warranties of any kind are declared or implied. Readers acknowledge that the author is not engaging in the rendering of legal, financial, medical or professional advice. The content within this book has been derived from various sources. Please consult a licensed professional before attempting any techniques outlined in this book.

By reading this document, the reader agrees that under no circumstances is the author responsible for any losses, direct or indirect, which are incurred as a result of the use of information contained within this document, including, but not limited to, — errors, omissions, or inaccuracies.

Table of Contents

Introduction

How efficient is hypnosis? That's the kind of question anyone considering hypnotherapy asks, and it interest researchers to hear this because it has been a point for decades.

The research seems to paint hypnotherapy a positive picture of effectiveness. Many studies have shown that hypnosis can result in long-term weight loss; hypnosis records higher success rates.

Research organized in 1985 is one of the first looks at weight loss hypnosis compared to two groups. A group worked on diet changes and began exercising; the other did the same thing but additionally receiving hypnotherapy. After about seven months and two years, the hypnosis group had sustained and increased weight loss while the other group had gained most of the weight back.

Correspondingly, a 1986 research work examined twenty women who were 20 percent overweight. After six months, the hypnosis team had lost 17 pounds, while the non-hypnotic team had just lost a half-pound.

A 1996 meta-evaluation observed the result of attaching hypnosis to weight loss treatments. What the researchers discovered was alarming and convincing. Hypnosis was almost twice the weight loss on treatment, and after the procedure, it dramatically increased its efficiency by 146 percent.

Recently, a 2014 study discovered that hypnosis had several options for a positive influence on weight loss. Those who participate in receiving hypnosis declined in weight, as well as enhanced their eating habits. The improved body structure was another benefit discovered in the study.

Are you ready to kick start your weight loss journey? To start, there are several options. Visiting a professional hypnotherapist physically for a session, or fix up a virtual conference with a hypnotherapist will be fine. All method as regards hypnosis has shown promising result for weight loss.

One-on-One Hypnosis - A hypnotherapist can assist you in recognizing the unconscious limitations that are holding your bond. Additionally, a hypnotherapist sees you through in those sessions to resolve the limitations. These are done in offices or better done via video conferencing.

Guided Hypnosis: A guided hypnosis record can help you quickly start and learn hypnosis mechanisms at your residence or on the go. More importantly, these are records from certified hypnotherapists who walk you through induction and then give positive suggestions through the recording.

Self-Hypnosis; engaging in self-hypnosis, individuals take on the responsibility of hypnotherapists, making use of a memorized script to lure them into hypnosis and, after that, deliver positive suggestions. Get lose from every habit and attain your weight loss targets.

Shut your eyes, visualize your food cravings going off, imagine a day of eating only what's best for you. Imagine hypnosis eventually helping you lose weight- because the news is; it does. Here are ten hypnotic suggestions to try straight away.

Several people have not realized that adding trance to your weight loss scheme can help you lose weight and keep it off further.

Hypnosis precedes calorie counting by a few centuries, but attention hasn't been given to the long-aged techniques, not embracing completely as an effective strategy of weight loss. Very recently, there has been a scant scientific proof to support the legitimate resolutions of respected hypnotherapists,

Even after the convincing and compelling mid-nineties evaluations of 18 hypnotic kinds of research, psychotherapy clients who learned self-hypnosis lost double as much weight as those who didn't. Hypnotherapy, therefore, has been a well-kept weight loss mystery.

Until hypnosis has happily forced you or someone you know to buy a new, smaller wardrobe, it may be not easy to be convinced that this mind-over technique could help you get a handle on eating.

Chapter 1   Hypnosis in General

All of us are familiar with the somewhat clichéd and stereotypical line, "You are slowly falling asleep" connected with hypnotism, right? This line leads us to believe that hypnosis is something 'bad' and a hypnotist can control us entirely during a hypnotic state. Similarly, you may have seen stage hypnosis when the phenomenon is said to be 'magical.'

However, in truth, like meditation, hypnosis is a useful self-development tool to live life more meaningfully and happily than before. Hypnosis can be noticed as a form of meditation to achieve a specific goal. Meditation and hypnosis are similar concepts because both are excellent tools to achieve a state of deep relaxation and concentration.

So, what is hypnosis? It is a mental state where you achieve supremely focused concentration, heightened suggestibility, and reduced peripheral awareness. Hypnosis is a real psychological experience that has multiple therapeutic uses in clinical practice. The process of hypnotism typically includes three distinct steps, namely:

- Hypnotic Induction - This is the process that is used to achieve hypnosis. Ideally, the person undergoing hypnosis is made to sit comfortably in a chair or lie down on a couch or bed with eyes closed. Controlled breathing techniques can also be used to enhance the feeling of comfort. A memorized script, tape recording, or a live hypnotherapist is used in hypnotic induction.

- Hypnotic State - This state is achieved after hypnotic induction. The hypnotic state represents a calm, focused state of mind with heightened awareness. In this state, the person in a hypnotic state feels physically and mentally relaxed.

- Hypnotic Suggestion - When the person reaches the hypnotic state, he or she is ready to receive hypnotic suggestions, created to replace automatic thoughts in the subconscious mind. Ideas can be formulated in different ways; the traditional methods involve tips given as direct commands to the subconscious mind. In Ericksonian hypnosis, metaphors are used to make suggestions. In the neuro-linguistic programming method, tips mimic the patient's thought patterns.

Trained experts employ a multitude of techniques to induce a hypnotic state in people. The power of suggestion is one of the primary reasons why hypnosis is used for relaxation, reduction of pain, and to bring about positive behavioral changes.

Hypnosis is also referred to as a hypnotic suggestion or hypnotherapy. Hypnotherapists combine soothing verbal repetitions and mental imagery to get patients into a trance-like state. When patients are totally and completely relaxed, therapists use suggestive messages to bring positive transformations in the person's mind under hypnosis.

Interestingly, research has proved that not all human beings are equally hypnotizable. Some people appear to be more open to suggestions and hypnotherapy than others. The 'hypnotizability' trait differs from person to person. Brain imaging techniques reveal that patterns in brain connectivity change in people who are responsive to hypnotherapy and those who are not.

Before we move on to understand hypnosis, it might make sense to know the differences between the various terms used in this field.

- Hypnosis - Also referred to as the hypnotic state, hypnosis is the highly focused and relaxed state of mind that is reached after being hypnotized.

- Hypnotism - The process of hypnotic induction used to achieve the hypnotic state is called hypnotism.

- Hypnotherapy - This term refers to the use of hypnosis and hypnotism as a therapeutic tool. Hypnotherapists are trained and qualified professionals who help people to achieve hypnosis-powered self-development goals.

The Truth About Hypnosis

Hypnosis was considered one of the most controversial and misunderstood methods of psychological therapy for a long time. Misconceptions and myths surrounding hypnotherapy are mostly based on hypnotism produced by stage artists and magicians. This is nothing but a theatrical performance and has nothing in common with hypnosis being used as psychological therapy.

In a hypnotic state, people appear to be more open to suggestions than in their normal state. Positive tips given to people during hypnosis are called "post-hypnotic suggestions." They do not take effect until the individual has emerged from the hypnotic state.

When they are in the hypnotic state, the suggestions given to people play a crucial role in the process of hypnotherapy. Direct tips to bring about positive changes are typically not responded to by people in the normal psychological state of mind. However, during hypnosis, it seems that suggestions make a 'backdoor' entry into the consciousness of the affected person. This place is believed to be the root of significant psychological or behavioral changes.

Another essential myth to be dismissed is that people under hypnosis are not in control of themselves. Nothing can be further from the truth. Hypnotized people are entirely in control of themselves and will not act or do anything objectionable or harmful to themselves or others.

For a person to undergo hypnotherapy for positive results, he or she must participate in the process voluntarily and must have the ability to be hypnotized. Highly hypnotizable people do not always benefit from hypnotherapy.

Moreover, hypnotherapy is not a one-session treatment where lasting changes can be expected. People typically have to undergo a series of procedures to reinforce constructive suggestions for positive changes repeatedly. The most general use of hypnotherapy is to break bad habits, recall and acknowledge past forgotten memories, overcome stress, anxiety, and insomnia, and manage pain.

History of Hypnosis

While stage hypnosis and its related 'magical' effects are relatively new, hypnosis has been in use in Western psychology for thousands of centuries. Eastern religions like Hinduism have self-hypnosis as part of their religious rituals. In the 11th century, Avicenna, a famed physician from Persia, is credited with documenting the concept of hypnotism.

One of the earliest forms of using hypnosis as a distinct therapy in the field of psychology is given to Franz Anton Mesmer, an 18th-century healer. Mesmer was a firm believer in astrological principles and opined that heavenly bodies directly influence human physical, emotional, and mental health.

Initially, Mesmer used magnets in grand, theatrical ways resulting in expected spasmodic muscular contractions, which, in turn, frequently resulting in curing of illnesses. Mesmer used rationalistic terms like magnetism and gravitation for his healing methods. He said that these healing methods could influence the subtle fluids within the human body. His methods and subsequent subsets established by others are collectively referred to as Mesmerism.

Even though Mesmer and his methods were discredited, later on, he was able to convince his followers that they can channelize their 'animal magnetism' to cure and alleviate the symptoms of their illnesses and ailments.

The earliest distinction between Mesmer's kind of 'mesmerism' and modern hypnotherapy was made by Dr. James Braid, a Manchester surgeon who coined the term 'hypnosis' in 1843. The word has its roots name of the Greek God of Sleep Hypnos because most forms of mesmerism involved a sleep-like status for the patient. Braid proposed that the reason for Mesmer's methods having some effect on followers was the suggestion's power.

Braid worked with hypnotherapy. In his early studies, he thought that hypnosis could result in a distinctive condition of the nervous system that could be suitable for suggestion-based cures. However, further studies made him reject his theory, and he emphasized the importance of "mental factors" playing a role in hypnotherapy.

However, the neural connection was not entirely dismissed. Ivan Pavlov, a prominent figure who contributed immensely to psychology, worked on the neural inhibition theory as part of his research on the physiology of sleep. Many of Pavlov's ideas have proven to be reasonably accurate in a general sense.

Jean Marie-Charcot was a French neurologist who started using hypnosis as a therapy to cure a disorder highly prevalent during her time, namely hysteria (which, in Greek, which translates to "wandering uterus"). Sigmund Freud studied this concept with Charcot. However, as he was not a very good hypnotist, he used this theory to reach patients' subconscious minds through free association.

Modern-day hypnotherapy was founded in the early 20th century by members of a society called "Nancy School of Hypnosis." The elaborate theories on hypnotic therapy proposed by the founding members of this group replaced many of the older ideas, including the neural connections and Braid's early theories based on magnetism and gravitation.

Freud also believed in the theories of the Nancy School, believing that people generally tend to repress painful and traumatic memories. He thought that hypnotherapy could help such people come to terms with these traumatic memories and cure mental and psychological problems rooted in the repressed and forgotten memories.

Other important psychologists who contributed to the field of hypnotherapy included Clark Hull (his 1933 discussion based on his research is still used by modern therapists and is considered a classic), Milton Erickson (whose name is most closely connected to clinical hypnosis today), and Jay Hayley (who developed the MRI Interactional Model of therapy). Neuro-Linguistic Programming (NLP) is one of the most famous forms of hypnotherapy used by therapists today.

The research on hypnotherapy continues, with people from all over the world reaping the benefits.

Common Misconceptions about Hypnosis

Hypnotists cannot make you do anything against your will. No, they cannot make you cluck like a hen or any such ridiculous thing. Instead, it is very similar to meditation and allows you to enter into a state of deep relaxation and concentration. The person undergoing hypnosis is in complete control of himself or herself. Here are some common misconceptions about hypnosis for your reference and better understanding:

You are unconscious or asleep - The deep state of relaxation and concentration is frequently mistaken for a state of unconsciousness or deep sleep. While the origin of the word is rooted in Hypnos, the Greek God of Sleep, in reality, you don't go to sleep. Under the influence of hypnosis, you are fully awake and are acutely aware of your surroundings and what is happening to you.

You lose control - This idea is a total myth. The person under hypnotic induction experiences a heightened level of concentration and focus. All distractions are tuned out, and he or she achieve total relaxation. The person under hypnosis can open his or her eyes at any time and is in complete control.

Hypnosis is a magic pill - Hypnosis does not promise to cure anything and everything. You should have a deep desire to make a positive difference in your life, and hypnotherapy is a device that will help you in attaining your desire. However, you have to work at it. Hypnosis is not a magic pill.

You can get stuck in a hypnotic state - Many movies depict scenes where the villain hypnotizes someone, and this person can never wake up at all because he or she remains hypnotized forever! This scene is only for fictional movies and does not happen in reality. In real life hypnosis sessions, you can open your eyes and come back to your surroundings anytime you want.

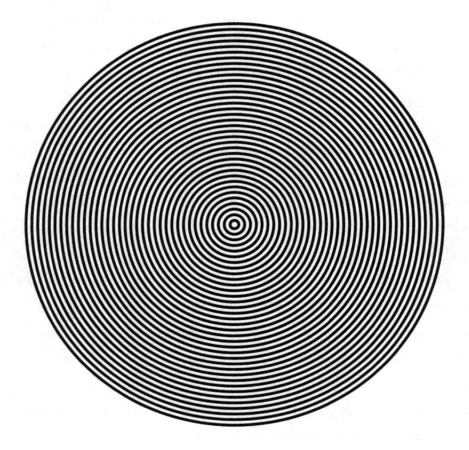

Chapter 2   Procedures

The Analytical Technique

Utilize a technique for unwinding

There are various approaches to start a logical treatment session (otherwise called creative mind treatment), yet it is essential to get the subject to a responsive state. Attempt to put them on a comfortable love seat/couch and close their eyes. At no time are they going to hit the hay?

Each time you converse with the point, utilize a smooth, calming tone. You can attempt to get them down from 100 gradually. You can intentionally and methodically tense them, hold them, and after that, discharge every one of their muscles for progressively anxious patients.

It can likewise work with controlled relaxing. The point puts his hands on his chest and abdomen—at times, the trance specialist can do this part—while the subject gradually inhales through his nose and mouth.

The visuals you need to utilize are focused on

When your subject is in a responsive state, you have to limit the imaging sets you're centering on. Insofar as you're wary, you can endeavor some energizing examinations. To draw a correspondingly typical response from the subject, select positive pictures, for example, an occasional party, graduation, a wedding, or a blend of different images in a grouping.

If they have to unwind, you can help them "construct" the photos with ideal sentiments and recollections from the point partners' attributes.

You may make them look for wonderful pictures to supplant horrendous ones on the off chance that you help an injury case.

Pick how to express these visuals.

There is a great deal of adaptability here, so it should be custom-made to your point's necessities and perhaps talked about before the session.

You can make the articulation mode part of the investigation with so much scope. Maybe having your theme drive their photos in a vehicle or making a film of their most joyful recollections would be something you can attempt. Possibly having the subject in their photos going on an undertaking could be a serious encounter to endeavor.

Locate an innovative method to emblematically dispose of antagonistic pictures, enabling the positive images to remain in the area. Consider something strict like tossing the poor photos in a trash can or anticipating them on a screen, so the lovely symbolism has space in the psyche.

Talk through the strategy to your theme.

Your subject is in a condition of gathering, yet not sleeping. You control them. Steer the photos of the subject a great way; however, take a gander at their responses on the off chance that they stand up. Keep the smooth, steady voice tone all through the session. Propose symbolism that blends with their instant responses positively. Be prepared in the event of a negative physical reaction to getting them out of the mesmerizing state.

Utilize a few gatherings

You may set aside some effort to discover what techniques and pictures work best with the theme for trial conditions. Also, neither trance inducer nor subject ought to anticipate a quick fix, especially in occurrences of injury or when managing expanded torment suffering. The sleep-inducing strategy can take numerous sessions from the earliest starting point.

Timetable intermittent session's time/interim. If the sessions don't function as they expect, the two sides should raise issues.

The Suggestion Technique

Put a proposition in the psyche of the subject.

This is a more direct strategy than the imaging method. This may viably require a proposition to utilize your creative mind. However, recommendations ought to appear to require less exertion if they are powerful.

This strategy can lead to conduct as well as recognition alterations that are more explicit than different techniques. It will require an increasingly exhaustive direction from the trance inducer.

After sleep-inducing enlistment, talk the guidance.

They are open to proposals after the theme is mesmerizing, and the trance inducer can travel through the guidance or condition. The advice must be specific, however simple. Make a signal for the beginning and closure of the effect of the guidance.

Try not to go astray during the molding from your quiet, consistent voice. Carry the subject with the signal you created from the proposal time frame.

Focus on a particular lead as well as inclination

It's ideal for endeavoring one recommendation at a minute in case you're testing. If your theme picks a specific point, they need to be evoked or stopped, change your bearings in like manner. The trance specialist can endeavor some useful recommendations in the test condition as long as they are wary not to hurt them. The trance specialist may endeavor to propose mediation.

The trance specialist may endeavor to get them to respond to an order or improvement, like playing a melodic note with one activity. The trance specialist may recommend something progressively mind-boggling— perhaps on the off chance that you give an order sentence, you may have them respond with a specific sentence.

Plan Meetings all the time

Even though this system isn't as drawn out as the imaging strategy, different sessions can also be useful in testing the trial rendition adequacy. It can likewise be valuable to broadened treatment sessions.

Keep up correspondence among trance specialist and subject to decide whether to lead or potentially a way of life are improved by treatment. Whenever broadened sessions don't affect, ensure that there is not any more serious medicinal issue.

Consider different systems. On the off chance that proposal treatment doesn't work, at that point, consolation might be required from the theme to seek after various procedures.

Look at the other sleep-inducing stunts/approaches for their potential advantages.

For example, picture and intellectual treatment. On the chance that they are set up to endeavor these different methods, talk about the subject. An emotional wellness expert ought to be counseled for further assessment if impressively increasingly articulated dysfunctional behavior is introducing itself.

Intellectual Techniques

Get ready for a more profound unwinding for your subject.

Since the intellectual treatment stunt, for the most part, includes investigating the mind's oblivious memory focuses and potentially expelling undesirable recollections/thinks, this will, in general, include a more profound daze like condition.

Other than the techniques for setting the subject in a casual state, it might be smart to dispose of all potential commotion contamination. Avoid potential risks to counteract the unsettling outer influence of the session.

Examine the destinations of the gatherings in detail

For test sessions, ensure that your point is good with you inspecting their subliminal. For therapeutic sessions, the subject may not explicitly recognize what thoughts or memories they need or need to be evacuated to explain as much as possible. In trial sessions, it will be up to the trance inducer on the off chance that they need to go in with warning of the foundation of the subject or enter dazzle—and not hazard predispositions as this is exploratory for the two sides.

In the case of managing a terrible memory or a wellspring of torment, it might be useful to get setting information when searching for the mind. Be as sensibly obliging as conceivable in transmitting these fundamental data to you to make the subject agreeable.

Through their recollections, talk about the theme.

The hypnotherapist will have a discussion with the musings of the subject during the session. The stupor like state sidesteps the conscious personality, so the trance specialist addresses the subliminal legitimately.

This empowers the subject to address another person about stuff that they may not typically uncover. During a spellbinding session, as individuals are as yet conscious, they will recollect that they uncover this memory to the trance specialist.

The trance inducer could endeavor a few techniques on the recollections of the subject in a trial session. The hypnotherapist could start with something essential like adolescence or later—perhaps at a vocation and discussion about the subject during that experience through their enthusiastic state.

The trance inducer will tune in to the relationship of the subject with these recollections during the test session and can connect from memory to memory and structure a picture of how the psyche of the subject functions at the intuitive level.

Other test systems may incorporate having the subject return to antiquated recollections to discover crisp things about the case that they had not understood.

In a remedial session, the trance inducer should manage the discussion to find the wellspring of the defective memory, pose inquiries to drive the patient toward this path, and smoothly decide why the mind causes the injury and additionally agony of the theme.

In the treatment session, in a perfect world, the patient will currently have the option to purposely confront as well as understand the issue recollections when the trance inducer removes the patient from the daze.

Know what the subjective hypnotherapy ought to be utilized for

Since this is a profound plunge into a subject's mind, the benefits of this strategy are various, yet ought to be intently focused likewise with different systems. This might be a private involvement with related dangers and rewards in this system's exploratory stunt variation.

With the subliminal specialist as their guide, the point may investigate obscure districts of their psyche. The two sides ought to build up that it is suitable to investigate the obscure recollections of the subject, and to be sure, an ideal outcome.

Employments of this treatment incorporate long-standing lightening concerns, nervousness, a sleeping disorder, discouragement, stress, sadness (from private misfortune), weight reduction, poor practices, and even certain physical conditions, for example, skin illnesses.

If you attempt different analyses or tending to various horrendous issues, only a couple for each session might be prudent.

On the chance that the circumstance of the subject compounds significantly as well as winds up unsafe to the point of damage—look for quick crisis medicinal consideration.

Have intermittent gatherings booked

Since this strategy might be less exact than the others, it might take a few endeavors to fathom how to get to the recollections of your subject for the intellectual stunt and become acclimated with the affiliations they commonly make. It might require some investment for injury situations to initially perceive and adapt to the issue recollections in a subject.

For test cases, as this is exploratory, you and the point should not want to stay on a particular topic or memory track.

In injury occasions, consider longer interims between sessions when dealing with particularly upsetting recollections/torment.

Talk about whether to keep a diary/record of any sort on what is examined in every session. This will keep track of the various courses that may lead your point through your exploratory stunts. In injury cases, a paper will help with the goal of disconnected recollections not raised again superfluously. Any memory might be related in startling ways; however, keep up as a top priority.

Ensure that the subject has a lot of time to rest when sessions since this technique need a more profound daze.

Audit this present procedure's results

Ensure that the theme reacts to this profound jump stunt, or different techniques ought to be considered. The logical or proposition feats might be increasingly viable if the intellectual methodology doesn't work.

The instance of the subject may have alluded to a progressively explicit therapist or specialist on the off chance that it is unreasonably genuine for any of these strategies.

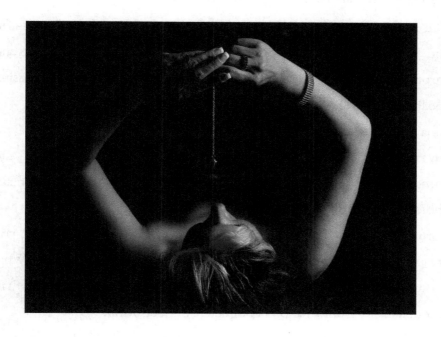

Chapter 3 How to Use Hypnosis to Transform and Reprogram your Mind

Using Hypnosis to Transform Your Mind

The idea of hypnotherapy brings out reactions ranging from "cross-arm and wary in dismay" to "shocked in unadulterated amazement and surprise." There is no denying the supernatural quality encompassing spellbinding; it stays to puzzle individuals' psyches.

As a result, we tend to live our lives amid a society in which the day to day rush of events doesn't leave us much time for thought and contemplation. This means that we are faced with making difficult choices in dealing with our happiness and well-being.

Fortunately, this idea is a long way from a reality of true to life when you grasp spellbinding. In this way, we have a much-improved idea. What about utilizing the incredible intensity of hypnotherapy rather than manufacturing a universe of a completely perfect world?

Since there is a persuading reason for hypnotherapy behind the cloak of wizardry and visual impairment, to fix our brains, bodies, and in the long run our universe.

As a general rule, trance has been utilized worldwide as an instrument for mending for in any event 4,000 years; however, science has just begun to reveal this entrancing riddle in recent years. Their outcomes hugely affect our ability to change our thoughts and convictions, conduct, and practices only as our recognition and reality improve things.

In any case, most importantly, science has discovered a solid reality: entrancing is valid. What's more, on the off chance you accept you've never had mesmerizing, take it again.

Hypnosis' characterizing practices are:

Increased suggestibility. Making musings progressively open and responsive.

It improved creative thinking—creation in the eye of our psyches of striking, frequently illusory symbolism.

Without thinking, discernment. Quieting the cognizant systems that create thoughts while improving passionate mindfulness.

These three characterizing highlights make spellbinding a particular and useful instrument for private transformation.

Many of the issues that unleash destruction on the globe today happen because we have significant mental wounds to which there has been no inclination.

We download information from the globe around us at lightning speed until we're around nine years old. During this minute, our subliminal feelings and practices are typically shaped — before we built up our balanced reasoning (got when our mind frames the prefrontal cortex).

In our childhood, for instance, someone can let us know, "you're ugly." At the time, our brains can't defend the likelihood that any individual who reveals to us this will have a crummy day or experience the ill effects of their psychological wounds. Instead, our energetic, honest personalities accept, "goodness, and I'm frightful." That works for "you're stunning" on a kinder note, just as some other great attestation. We are importance making machines in this incredibly porous minute in our life.

We quickly credit importance to them when certain events happen in our youthfulness. What produces our subliminal convictions is that allotted significance.

This is the place hypnotherapy comes in. Nothing fixes these significantly established enthusiastic wounds more rapidly than the hypnotherapy prescription. We have discovered that, in the condition of mesmerizing, we can get to and interface legitimately with these intuitive zones of our psyche— without our ordinary cognizant reasoning.

During trance, a trance inducer controls their patients back to their youth's zenith occasions. The patient can reassign centrality to them once recollections of the case are gotten to.

Reprogramming your Mind through Hypnosis

Your intuitive personality has an enormous impact on dealing with your background— from the sorts of sustenance you eat to the exercises you take each day, the income level you get, and even how you react to unpleasant conditions.

Your intuitive feelings and understandings manage all of it. In a nutshell, your subliminal personality resembles an airplane's auto-pilot work. Following a particular way has been pre-modified, and you cannot go astray from that course except if you initially change the customized guidelines.

The "intuitive" is your mind's part that works underneath your customary arousing cognizance level. At this moment, you are primarily utilizing your cognizant personality to peruse these expressions and retain their centrality. However, your subliminal personality works hectically in the background, absorbing, or dismissing information dependent on a present perspective on the globe around you. When you were a tyke, this current observation began to shape. Your intuitive personality drenches like wipe data with each experience.

While you were youthful, your consciousness rejected nothing since you had no prior perspectives that would negate what it saw. It merely recognized that it was genuine every one of the information you acquired during your initial puberty. You can almost certainly observe why this sometime down the road turns into an issue. Each time you were called by somebody stupid, useless, slow, apathetic, or more terrible, your subliminal personality put away the information for reference.

You may likewise have messages about your life potential or requirements relying upon your physical aptitudes, the shade of the skin, sex, or money related status. By the minute you were 7 or 8 years of age, you had a solid premise of religion on all the programming you viewed from people in your lives, network shows, and other natural impacts. Since you are developed, you may figure you can dispose of the negative or false messages you've consumed in your initial life. However, it isn't so necessary. Keep in mind this information is put away underneath your conscious awareness level. The first minute you understand this is the point at which it constrains your advancement in building an actual existence that is adjusted, prosperous, and gainful.

Have you, at any point, endeavored to arrive at a target and consistently undermined yourself? Goading, right? It is fundamental to comprehend that regardless of what you do, you are not flawed or destined to come up short. You are bound to have some old, customized messages that contention with the new conditions that you need to make. This is incredible news since it suggests that on the off chance that you first set aside the effort to reconstruct your intuitive personality, you can achieve pretty much anything! Before we discover how to rebuild your psyche, it's fundamental to comprehend that the programming proceeds right up 'til today. You draw certain discoveries with each experience you have and store the messages that will direct your future conduct.

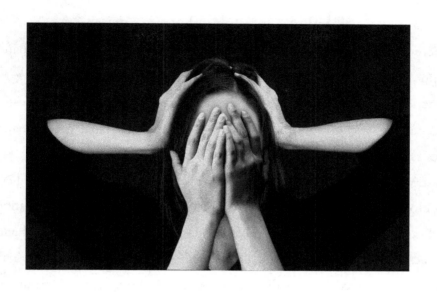

Chapter 4   Gastric Band Hypnosis for Weight Loss

There is another procedure for weight loss known as gastric band hypnosis that has been created over the recent years. It is coming to America from the UK and Europe, and there are a few preliminaries in progress to test how well Americans react to the virtual gastric band process.

Gastric band hypnosis utilizes the creative mind instead of the surgical tool to assist overweight with peopling to recover power over their eating and movement practices. You most likely recognize what the gastric band medical procedures or weight loss medical procedures include. The technique is acted in a medical clinic working room where a group of specialists and attendants make little entry points in your chest and stomach and slip small careful instruments and cameras into your internal body. They cut and consume a passage around your stomach and join a banding gadget that an area off your stomach's top piece. The size of this top piece of your stomach can be balanced with the goal that it tends to be made to get just a limited quantity of nourishment. So, you become truly unequipped for eating more than 4 or 5 pieces quickly.

When this particular activity is performed, if you somehow manage to eat beyond what your new littler stomach can hold, you will be genuinely weakened. This is a typical outcome that is classified as "dumping." It is regular to such an extent that a word was conceived to portray the marvel. The purpose behind the surgery is to make it compulsory for you to eat littler measures of nourishment. Littler meals will mean more noteworthy weight loss. There is no assurance that you will eat littler meals, regardless of whether you have the activity. Furthermore, there are times when the individuals who have had the activity have overeaten and messed more up to themselves because their inner organs were changed.

This new weight loss program, gastric band hypnosis, benefits from the symbolism of the surgery. Utilizing your creative mind, you will be persuaded that you have had the band embedded, and you will react as though you have had the activity. Your mind is a beneficial asset for change, and your creative mind is the way into your disappointments and your victories. Anything that you can envision enough, your body will react as though it is valid.

By utilizing the intensity of your mind, your stomach will feel littler, and you will subsequently wind up eating littler measures of nourishment. The program is additionally intended to manage and work through the reasons that you have eaten a lot previously. Regardless of whether those reasons are propensities or feelings, your explanations behind overeating will vanish. I am leaving you with the capacity to assemble the new tendencies that will continue your new, more advantageous life for an amazing remainder.

A couple of TV programs broadcast reports about a type of mental gastric band medical procedures. This is not surgery at everything except an inventive method for utilizing your creative mind to enable your body to envision that you had the surgery. Also, since your body envisions that your stomach has dried, you currently react with feeling full speedier and declining to eat an excessive amount of nourishment.

This seems like an outlandish idea to numerous overweight individuals, such as yourself, who have battled for so long to evacuate the abundance weight. If you see how our minds work, however, it doesn't appear to be so outlandish. Take, for instance, how we react in the present to things that we have comparable encounters to before.

Music is something that a considerable lot of us tune in to consistently. What's more, since music is something that goes all through style, we most likely had tuned in to specific forms of music and particular melodies when we were a lot more youthful than we tune in to today. The sentiments and encounters we experienced at that younger age are most likely only ancient histories for us today. However, all the time, when you tune in to an old tune today, it can have the impact of taking you back to the emotions, musings, and occasions of your life from quite a while in the past. So, you know how exceptionally ground-breaking your creative mind is.

Shouldn't something be said about an encounter that you have never had? By what method can your mind make impressions that you have no earlier information on experiencing? Indeed, we do have specific thoughts of what things would feel like, or how we would react to particular circumstances dependent on comparable events that we have experienced. We probably won't know how it feels to fly since a large portion of us I can securely say have never flu assisted by some airplane. Furthermore, if you have ever observed, you likely envisioned that you could fly yourself. What's more, if you utilize your creative mind, you may ultimately have had the option to truly feel like you were flying during that fantasy or dream.

So, you see, regardless of whether you have never had an encounter, you can, in any case, envision what it would feel like if you did. When you orchestrate to utilize gastric band hypnosis to help you re-deal with your eating and build up another more beneficial connection with nourishment, you increase an incredible partner for your weight loss.

Gastric Band Surgery Versus Gastric Band Hypnosis

So, you're considering quitting any funny business about your weight issue. You feel genuinely in the wrong way, and you need to begin thinning down. You are so genuine that you are currently in any event, considering surgery to help you in dropping the weight. Since we realize that you are not kidding, we should go over your choices.

Weight loss includes taking in smaller calories than you expend. If you eat 3500 calories in seven days, you typically will convert into you losing 1 pound of weight. That implies that you will need to dispense with 500 calories per day to get that going. Through the span of a year, you will have shed 50 pounds. Increment the measure of calories you dispense with from your day by day or week after week diet, and you will build the number of pounds you lose over the long run. Those are the essentials of weight loss, and those nuts and bolts don't change in any event, when you pick surgery to help you in your weight loss venture.

Your surgery alternatives incorporate a few distinct systems, and the one that this article is concentrating on is the gastric band surgery. With gastric band surgery, you will be wheeled into the working room where you will be calmed, and a group of specialists will play out a laparoscopic surgery. This necessitates various little entry points that will be made in your chest and stomach region. Into these cuts, the specialists will embed small cameras and careful instruments. While watching their advancement on a TV screen, the specialists will have the option to remove areas of fat and push aside the organs encompassing your stomach. This is so they can make a passage underneath your stomach sack.

When that passage is made, the specialist will, at that point, introduce a band around the highest point of your stomach. This band is like a wind conclusion for your waste sack. This conclusion's motivation is to segregate the top piece of your stomach and utilize that to make a little store to catch the nourishment that you eat. It will, at that point, enter the remainder of your stomach gradually as it is separated and ready to course through that now little opening made by the gastric band.

After your gastric band is introduced, you will, in any case, need to eat littler measures of nourishment with the goal for you to get more fit. Recollect that the recipe for losing a pound seven days is to eat 500 fewer calories daily. That has not changed. What has changed is that your stomach is presently incapable of dealing with especially nourishment at once. Your stomach has indeed altered to be the size of a golf ball. Eating more than 4 or 5 pieces of food will currently put significant weight on your stomach related framework. You will have a downright awful physical reaction to consuming an excess of food. This is called dumping by specialists.

Gastric band hypnosis is a method for utilizing your creative mind in an exceptionally significant manner. When you use the gastric band hypnosis strategy, you will have a psychological gastric band introduced, and you will be guided to follow the littler bits program that the care patients would follow. Some virtual gastric band members locate that after the virtual gastric band is introduced, they feel a snugness in their stomachs. They determine the same sort of emotions from if they had particular careful activity performed. At the point when that occurs for you, you will, at that point, be affected to follow an eating program that comprises of less nourishment, and you will get thinner.

Corpulence is at an unprecedented high. In only us, the Centers for Disease Control and Prevention gauges that over 37% of the US populace is fat. That is more than 90 million grown-ups, and youngsters and the numbers continue expanding a long time after year. The expansion in stoutness levels has likewise prompted more individuals to investigate gastric band surgery to lose a great deal of weight rapidly. Even though this sort of operation works, it's not without complexities. It is obtrusive surgery that requires joining a band that makes your stomach about 90% littler. The outcome is you eat significantly less nourishment and shed pounds bit by bit after some time. This surgery is a genuinely necessary lifesaver in case you're severely overweight. If you don't lose weight, you could wind up doing combating hazardous sicknesses, including hypertension, coronary illness, and diabetes.

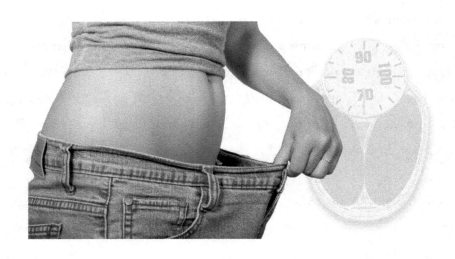

Chapter 5   Guided Hypnosis for Weight Loss

Even if hypnosis has no physical side effects, it must be done well and by a certified hypnotist for it to be effective. There are many hypnotists in the market, but getting the right one is a challenge. We shall give you a guide into getting an excellent hypnotist to help in your weight loss journey. We shall also discuss various apps that use hypnosis to aid in weight loss and a guide to losing weight through hypnotherapy.

Step by Step Guide to Hypnotherapy for Weight Loss

1. Believe. A significant part of the intensity of spellbinding lies in your conviction that you have a method for assuming responsibility for your desires. If you don't figure entrancing will enable you to change your emotions, it will probably have little impact.

2. Become agreeable. Go to a spot where you may not be stressed. This can resemble your bed, a couch, or an agreeable, comfortable chair anyplace. Ensure you bolster your head and neck. Wear loose garments and ensure the temperature is set at an agreeable level. It might be simpler to unwind if you play some delicate music while mesmerizing yourself, particularly something instrumental.

3. Focus on an item. Discover something to take a gander at and focus on in the room, ideally something somewhat above you. Utilize your concentration for clearing your leader of all contemplations on this item. Make this article the main thing that you know.

4. Breathing is crucial. When you close your eyes, inhale profoundly. Reveal to yourself the greatness of your eyelids and let them fall delicately. Inhale profoundly with an ordinary mood as your eyes close. Concentrate on your breathing, enabling it to assume control over your

whole personality, much like the item you've been taking a gander at previously. Feel progressively loose with each fresh breath. Envision that your muscles disperse all the pressure and stress. Permit this inclination from your face, your chest, your arms, lastly, your legs to descend your body. When you're entirely loose, your psyche should be clear, and you will be a self-mesmerizing piece.

5. Display a pendulum. Customarily, the development of a swing moving to and from has been utilized to energize the center is spellbinding. Picture this pendulum in your psyche, moving to and fro. Concentrate on it as you unwind to help clear your brain.

6. Start by focusing on 10 to 1 in your mind. You advise yourself as you check down that you are steadily getting further into entrancing. State, "10, I'm alleviating. 9, I get increasingly loose. 8. I can feel my body spreading unwinding. 7, Nothing yet unwinding I can handle.... 1, I'm resting profoundly. Keep in mind that you will be in a condition of spellbinding when you accomplish one all through.

7. Waking up from self-hypnosis. Once during spellbinding, you have accomplished what you need, you should wake up. From 1 to 10, check back. State in your mind: "1, I wake up. 2, I'll feel like I woke up from a significant rest when I tally down. 3, I think wakeful more.... 10, I'm wakeful, I'm new.

8. Develop a plan. Reinventing your mind with spellbinding requires consistent redundancy. You ought to endeavor in a condition of spellbinding to go through around twenty minutes per day. While beneath, shift back and forth between portions of the underneath referenced methodologies. Attempt to assault your poor eating rehearses from any edge.

9. Learn to refrain from emotional overeating. One of the main things you should endeavor to do under mesmerizing is to influence yourself. You are not intrigued by the frightful nibble of food you experience issues kicking. Pick something that you will, in general, revel in like frozen yogurt. State "Dessert tastes poor and makes me feel debilitated." Repeat twenty minutes until you're prepared to wake up from the trance. Keep in mind; excellent eating regimen doesn't suggest you have to quit eating, simply eat less awful sustenance. Simply influence yourself to devour less food, you know, is undesirable.

10. Write your very own positive mantra. Self-spellbinding ought to likewise be utilized to reinforce your longing to eat better. Compose a mantra to rehash in a trance state. It harms me and my body when I overeat.

11. Imagine the best thing for you. Picture what you might want to be more beneficial to support your longing to live better. From when you were slenderer, take a picture of yourself or do your most extreme to figure what you'd resemble in the wake of shedding pounds. Concentrate on this image under mesmerizing. Envision the trust you'd feel on the off chance that you'd be more advantageous. This will cause you to comprehend that when you wake up. Eat each supper with protein. Protein is especially valuable at topping you off and can improve your digestion since it advances muscle improvement. Fish, lean meat, eggs, yogurt, nuts, and beans are great wellsprings of protein. A steak each dinner might be counterproductive, yet if you're eager, eating on nuts could go far to helping you accomplish your objectives.

12. Eat a few, modest meals daily. If you don't eat for quite a while, your digestion will go down, and you will stop fat consuming. If you expend

something modest once every three or four hours, your metabolism will go up, and when you plunk down for dinner, you will be less hungry.

13. Eat organically grown foods. You will be loaded up with foods grown from the ground and furnish you with supplements without putting any pounds on. To start shedding pounds, nibble on bananas rather than treats to quicken weight reduction.

14. Cut down on unhealthy fats. It tends to be helpful for you to have unsaturated fats, similar to those in olive oil. Nonetheless, you should endeavor to limit your saturated fat and trans-fat intake. Both of these are significant factors that add to coronary illness.

15. Learn more about healthy cooking. In preparing meals, trans fats are common, mainly when eating meals, sweets, and fast food.

Saturated fats may not be as bad as trans fats. However, they might be undesirable. Primary saturated fat sources include spreads, cheddar cheese, grease, red meat, and milk. The journey to weight loss is not an easy one. A person needs a lot of help and motivation to succeed. With the help of hypnotherapy, one can easily stay the course and watch the pounds melt away. Following the guide above and with a credible hypnotherapist or mastering self-hypnosis will help you achieve your goals.

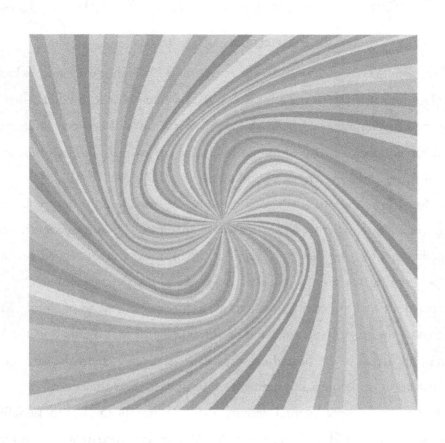

Chapter 6 Advantages of Weight Loss Meditation

Still, wondered why people are meditating? Which difference, which value does it bring to their lives? I was at a low point in my life when I started meditating and crying about my friend's loss. I started meditating on my counselor's suggestions to help ease my worries and continue my well-being and core strength building cycle.

A lot of people have various reasons to meditate. When you are contemplating, what was your reason to meditate? To an outsider, if you meditate, what they see you do is sit down, maybe cross-legged on the floor, staring at a point in the distance or sit with your eyes closed.

How does this, practicing meditation, influence your state of mind? Yet most of my students in yoga and meditation swear that meditation for 15 minutes a day is the best thing they can do to give them the strength, motivation, and compassion they need to do whatever they need.

Meditation is some mental activity that has significant health benefits both for the mind and the body. Meditation can help relax the mind, establish a more concentrated state, and enhance the brain's functioning.

Medical evidence suggests that meditation practice appears to elicit a level of physiological relaxation: decreases in blood pressure, slower heartbeats and faster breathing, and other biochemical improvements can occur as well.

1. This reduces the effects of many chronic illnesses, such as heart disease, cancer, and diabetes.
2. It helps and soothes chronic pain, anxiety, and migraine.

3. Meditation helps improve the role of the immune system and also prevents binge eating.

4. The asthma attacks offer considerable relief.

5. Reduces lactate in the blood, minimizing depression and anxiety.

6. Meditation has been documented to also help in lowering cholesterol.

7. Reduces muscle tension, and the nervous system is relaxed.

8. It assists in building self-confidence.

9. It helps monitor and aggressive mind.

10. Increases synchronization between brain waves.

11. Removing unhealthy habits helps.

12. Assists in the creation of intuition, imagination, and concentration.

13. It improves the ability to remember and enhances memory retention.

14. Enhances sleep habits and assists in eradicating insomnia

Meditation is the process of thought intensely for a while or relaxing one's mind. This can be done in silence or with the assistance of singing and is done for various reasons, ranging among religious or spiritual motives to a way to induce relaxation.

Meditation has in recent years grown in popularity in our modern, eventful world as a way to relieve stress. It has also emerged scientific evidence that meditation can be a valuable tool in the fight against chronic diseases, including depression, heart disease, and chronic pain.

Why can I remain motivated to lose weight?

The most critical aspect of creating constant and virtually infinite inspiration is linked with all the reasons you want to lose weight.

Keep in mind the broader sense of weight loss for you, like your health needs or how it can positively affect you every day, and the people around you, such as your family and close friends.

Focus on clear, observable, achievable, timely, and practical objectives. Make short but attainable goals first to find enjoyment and fulfillment in constant progress towards achieving long-term weight loss goals.

Have a clear, rational mind of not being too easy or too hard on yourself to reach the objectives by keeping the confidence and frustrations going far away.

Find people around you with the same drive as you do, and you are always encouraged and challenged to continue pushing for similar goals.

When you can keep these continually in mind, you can find that you will feel more motivated and determined to work through obstacles and circumstances toward achieving your long-term goals.

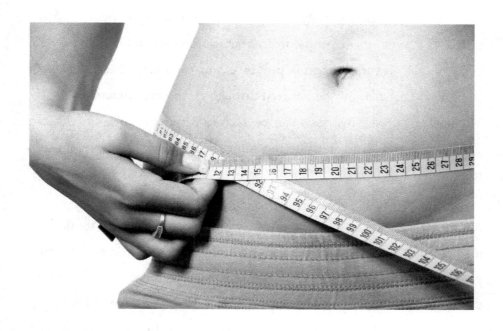

Chapter 7　How to Practice Everyday

When it becomes regular, it's so simple and so challenging. It's simple because 10-20 minutes a day is not much. It's difficult because many obstacles prevent most people from practicing regular meditation or self-hypnosis. However, conscious presence and calm responses instead of angry reactions can only be ensured through continuous practice.

Meditation and self-hypnosis can be seen as a diet or workout: we start with great enthusiasm initially, but after the first few days, we get into trouble.

What misconceptions are preventing this from happening?

Many people confuse meditation with relaxation and think that meditation is useful if you relax immediately. Lying on the ground after yoga and relaxing is not meditation but mere relaxation. In this case, we can systematically release stress through muscle relaxation and breathing. This is what we call fixation: when we strive to achieve a specific goal, regardless of the underlying situation. In meditation, however, we do not try to change the present case.

Let's take a general example: after a stressful day, we sit down to meditate. Usually, we don't feel like we can relax, and it is easy to concentrate on our breathing, no matter how much we try.

If we practice a fixative method, we can easily experience failure. Meditation teaches us that stressful and scattered conditions are part of life and that the first thing we can do about it is a curious observation. After all, meditation prepares us to flow with the ups and downs in our daily lives. Many times, there is no solution to a problem in the present situation, but we spend a deal of time and energy trying to find it, which can easily lead to even more stress.

Another misbelief is that while meditating, we shouldn't have thoughts. I always smile at this. We are thinking beings, and every day 60,000-125,000 impressions pass through our heads. Thanks to our thoughts, we can develop things; thanks to them, we can solve problems, create, and imagine things. When we talk about wanting to clear our minds because we overthink, we mean the thoughts that lead to anxiety. The purpose of meditation practice is to recognize our feelings, especially those that are continually talking and unconsciously controlling our subconscious. During meditation, we decide which thoughts we give and act upon, and which ones we let go. We don't want to exclude our dreams, but to develop a wiser relationship with them. So, it's not a problem if they do appear. We greet them and give them a name and then return to breathing. And when they come back more than once, we observe what emotions are beneath them.

Many people expect meditation to be an exciting trip. However, during meditation, we observe quite ordinary things: the flow of breath, the rising and falling of the belly, the sounds of our breathing, tingling, or lack of it in our toes. These may seem like annoying things, and for this reason, one of the first experiences you may have is that of a dull meditation session.

However, boredom stems from judgment, if we say something is not exciting, we think about that and avoid focusing on direct experience, which is the essence of meditation.

The next time you experience boredom, be aware of how you feel and observe how bored you are. What thoughts are passing through your mind? Ask yourself if you can release them so you can return to breathing.

We also expect that meditation must be something. Once you release that expectation, it becomes easier to practice. Releasing the urge to change also helps you practice not to qualify and judge everything, which is the essence of mindfulness meditation. If you have released all your misconceptions about meditation, let's jump into practice! Let me give you some useful tips for your meditation and self-hypnosis exercises.

Wear comfortable clothes. One of the main purposes of meditation is to relax the mind by preventing potential distractions. However, it will not be easy to relax if you feel uncomfortable with clothes that are too tight. During meditation practice, opt for soft garments and take off your shoes. If you plan to meditate in a cool place, wear a sweater or a cardigan.

Pick a peaceful room because you should practice meditation in a quiet place. In this way, you can concentrate solely on the exercise, away from outside distractions and stimulation. Search for a place where you don't run the risk of being interrupted while you are exercising.

For beginners, it is crucial to avoid any distractions. Turn off the TV, phone, and any other device that makes noise. If you want to put music in the background, choose something relaxing not to compromise concentration. If you prefer, you can listen to white noise or a sound of nature. The sound of a car or the barking of a dog shouldn't affect the success of the meditation. An essential element of this practice is to be aware of the surrounding noises without allowing them to take over the mind.

Many people believe it is beneficial to meditate outside. Unless you sit near a busy road or an unbearable noise source, you will be able to find peace under a tree or sit on a corner of grass in your favorite park.

Stretch a little before you start to avoid tightening up. During meditation, you will need to sit for a specified duration, so before starting, it is essential to relieving any muscle tension. A couple of minutes of stretching will help you prepare your body and mind. Moreover, it will prevent you from focusing on any minor pains, allowing you to relax. Remember to stretch your shoulder and neck muscles, especially if you have been sitting in front of the computer for a long time. Stretch the leg muscles, especially those in the inner thigh, to facilitate meditation in the lotus position. If you can't stretch your body muscles, consider using some other methods before meditation. Many specialists advise practicing some yoga exercises before starting to meditate.

Before starting, determine how long the session should last. Even though many masters suggest two sittings a day for 20 minutes, beginners can start with 5 minutes a day. Once you have decided the length, try to respect it. Don't be intimidated if you have the impression that it is not sufficient. It will take time and exercise to get the most out of meditation practice. In the beginning, the most important thing is to keep trying. Schedule an alarm clock by choosing a nice tune to know when the time is up.

Identify the goals you want to achieve with meditation or hypnosis. If you are doing this to reach a serious goal like weight loss, prepare a list of affirmation statements. Remember that you must say your affirmations concurrently: "I am eating healthy. I am losing weight. My clothes are fitting great, and I feel great." These are statements that you will recite to yourself when you are under hypnosis.

At this point, you can use the visualization in the way you prefer. Think of orange and cut it in half in your mind. Imagine squeezing the juice and feeling it on your fingers. Put it in your mouth. What is your reaction? What perceptions of taste and smell do you think? Then, move on to more meaningful visions. Imagine losing weight. Add as many details as possible. Always involve the five senses.

Try to understand that no meditation, self-hypnosis, affirmation or mantra will manifest in real life if you don't want it deep inside. For it to be effective, you should believe in yourself and your actions.

If it doesn't seem useful the first time, don't encourage yourself. Try again after a few days and revisit the experiences. You might be surprised. Open your mind. You must believe that there is a possibility that it works. Any skepticism on your part will hinder your progress.

Writing your suggestions before induction can be beneficial, as a visual list of what you want to work on can sometimes be more comfortable to retain than carefully assembled thoughts.

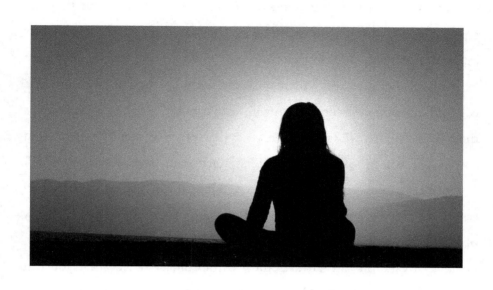

Chapter 8   Positive Affirmation for Weight Loss

Positive affirmations are ground-breaking proclamations that we rehash to ourselves (either in our mind or so anyone can hear), and they are typically things that we need to occur. They are utilized to improve our internal reasoning and impact our conduct and the achievement we experience. Let's assume them usually with conviction and genuine conviction; your subliminal brain will, at that point, come to acknowledge them as real. This will strengthen your new positive mental self-portrait and accuse you up of positive vitality. When your psyche starts to think something is valid, your disposition, conduct, and thinking will change to realize a perpetual change. Positive confirmations can be adjusted to any objective you wish to accomplish, including getting more fit.

Positive attestations are an extremely extraordinary device that you can use to assist you with shedding pounds. It very well may be trying under the most favorable circumstances when you are attempting to get more fit, particularly when you have melancholy, or you don't feel that great about yourself. Being overweight can cause a wide range of negative feelings that make it harder to remain spurred. Whatever you state to yourself significantly affects your circumstances and conditions. Truly the vast majority have no clue exactly how negative their idea designs are; have you ever gotten a brief look at your body in the mirror and felt your heart sink? Shouldn't something be said about when you state 'I'm so fat and disturbing?'

These are both extremely typical instances of negative self-talk. Negative self-talk is a deadly inspiration critic just as being exceptionally terrible for your general confidence. Getting thinner takes persistence and duty, and if you need to succeed long haul, you deserve to take the necessary steps to remain positive and persuaded. So what precisely are attestations? They are specific announcements composed or spoken in the current state that emphasizes the result or objective you need to accomplish.

The initial step to utilizing positive confirmations is to consider what you need to accomplish, and afterward develop various articulations that mirror this objective as though it were going on the present moment. For instance, if getting more fit is your objective, you may state, 'I effectively accomplish and keep up my optimal weight.' Or you may say 'I love and regard my body.' Here are some metal instances of positive confirmations for weight reduction:

· I effectively reach and keep up my optimal weight;

· I love and care for my body;

· I have the right to have a thin, healthy, alluring body;

· I love to practice consistently

· Everything I eat adds to my wellbeing and prosperity;

· I eat just when I am ravenous;

· I currently obviously observe myself at my optimal weight;

Weight reduction can appear to be difficult; utilizing weight reduction certifications to help you in the process can make it simpler. How about we feel free to survey this gigantic rundown to assist you with your weight reduction venture?

· Losing weight falls into place without a hitch for me.

· I am cheerfully accomplishing my weight reduction objectives.

· I am getting in shape each day.

· I love to practice normally.

- I am eating foods that add to my wellbeing and prosperity.
- I eat just when I am ravenous.
- I now unmistakably observe myself at my optimal weight.
- I love the flavor of sound nourishment.
- I am in charge of the amount I eat.
- I am getting a charge out of working out; it causes me to feel great.
- I am turning out to be fitter and more grounded regularly through exercise.
- I am effectively reaching and keep up my optimal weight
- I love and care for my body.
- I have the right to have a thin, healthy, appealing body.
- I am growing increasingly good dieting propensities constantly.
- I am getting slimmer consistently.
- I look and feel extraordinary.
- I take the necessary steps to be healthy.
- I am joyfully re-imagined achievement.
- I decide to work out.
- I need to eat foods that cause me to look and to feel great.
- I am liable for my wellbeing.
- I love my body.
- I am tolerant of making my better body.
- I am joyfully practicing each morning when I wake up with the goal that I can arrive at the weight reduction that I have needed.
- I am investing in my get-healthy plan by changing my dietary patterns from unfortunate to sound.
- I am content with each part I do in my extraordinary exertion to get more fit.

· Every day, I am getting slimmer and more beneficial.

· I am building up an alluring body.

· I am building up a way of life of energetic wellbeing.

· I am making a body that I like and appreciate.

Positive Affirmations for Losing Weight

· My way of life eating changes is changing my body.

· I am feeling extraordinary since I have lost more than 10 pounds in about a month and can hardly wait to meet my woman companion.

· I have a level stomach.

· I praise my capacity to settle on decisions around nourishment.

· I am cheerfully gauging 20 pounds less.

· I am adoring strolling 3 to 4 times each week and do conditioning practices, at any rate, three times each week

· I drink eight glasses of water a day.

· I eat foods grown from the ground day by day and eat, for the most part, chicken and fish.

· I am learning and utilizing the psychological, passionate, and otherworldly abilities for progress. I will change it!

· I will make new contemplations about myself and my body.

· I cherish and value my body.

· It's energizing to find my special nourishment and exercise framework for weight reduction.

· I am a weight reduction example of overcoming adversity.

· I am charmed to be the perfect load for me.

· It's simple for me to follow a solid nourishment plan.

· I decided to grasp the musings of trust in my capacity to roll out positive improvements throughout my life.

· It feels great to move my body. Exercise is enjoyable!

· I utilize profound breathing to assist me with unwinding and handle the pressure.

· I am a delightful individual.

· I have the right to be at my optimal weight.

· I am an adorable individual. I merit love. It is ok for me to shed pounds.

· I am a solid nearness on the planet at my lower weight.

· I discharge the need to scrutinize my body.

· I acknowledge and make the most of my sexuality. It's OK to feel erotic.

· My digestion is astounding.

· I keep up my body with ideal wellbeing.

These weight reduction confirmations will assist you with moving your excursion towards getting in shape. I trust these 50 weight-reduction certifications proved to be useful.

When you have made your positive assertions, you have to put aside time aside to rehearse them. You may pick one articulation and state it for all to hear multiple times toward the beginning of the day and numerous times at night, or you should rehash it to yourself as you consider it for the day. As you repeat your announcement, envision it occurring presently: See yourself doing or feeling the quintessence of what your confirmation is stating. Make it as genuine as conceivable in your inner consciousness. As you picture and envision your objective, your intuitive makes a psychological diagram.

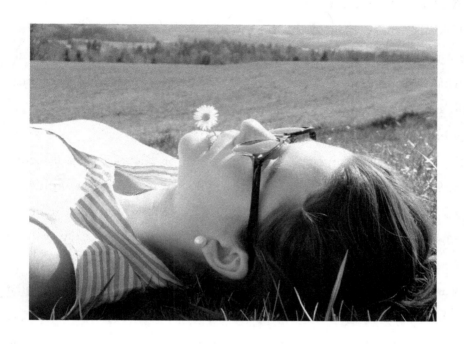

Chapter 9   Blasting Calories

We have all heard the word "calorie" and its relation to our body weight. Calories are contained in the foods we consume and are often misunderstood about how they affect us. In this topic, we seek to explain what they are, how to count them, and the best methods of blasting them to avoid weight gain.

What Are Calories, And How Do They Affect Your Weight?

A calorie is a fundamental estimating unit. For example, we use meters when communicating separation;' Usain Bolt went 100 meters in merely 9.5 seconds.' There are two units in this expression. One is a meter (a range unit), and the other is "second" (a period unit). Necessarily, calories are additional units of substantial amount estimation.

Many assume that a calorie is the weight measure (since it is often connected with an individual's weight). That is not precise, however. A calorie is a vitality unit (estimation). One calorie is proportional to the vitality expected to build the temperature by 1 degree Celsius to 1 kilogram of water.

Two particular sorts of calories come in: small calories and massive calories. Huge calories are the word connected to sustenance items.

You've likely observed much stuff on parcels (chocolates, potato chips, and so forth.) with' calorie scores.' Imagine the calorie score an incentive for a thing being' 100 cal.' this infers when you eat it. You will pick up about as much vitality (even though the calorie worth expressed and the amount you take advantage of it is never the equivalent).

All we eat has a particular calorie tally; it is the proportion of the vitality we eat in the substance bonds. B

These are mostly things we eat: starches, proteins, and fats. How about we take a gander at what number of calories 1 gram comprises of these medications: 1. Sugars 4 calories 2. Protein–3 calories. Fat–nine calories

Are my calories awful?

That is fundamentally equivalent to mentioning, "Is vitality awful for me?" Every single activity the body completes needs vitality. Everything takes energy to stand, walk, run, sit, and even eat. In case you're doing any of these tasks, it suggests you're utilizing vitality, which mostly infers you're' consuming' calories, explicitly the calories that entered your body when you were eating some nourishment.

To sum things up, for you, NO... calories are not terrible.

Equalization is the way to find harmony between the number of calories you devour and the number of calories you consume. On the chance that you eat fewer calories and spend more, you will become dainty. On the opposite side, on the possibility that you gobble up heaps of calories; however, you are a habitually lazy person; you will, in the long run, become stout at last.

Each movement we do throughout a day will bring about sure calories being spent. Here is a little rundown of the absolute most of the time performed exercises, just like the number of calories consumed.

Step by Step Instructions to Count Calories

You have to expend fewer calories than you consume to get thinner.

This clamor is simple in principle. It may be hard to deal with your nourishment admission in the contemporary sustenance setting. Calorie checking is one approach to address this issue and is much of the time used to get more fit. Hearing that calories don't make a difference is very common, and tallying calories is an exercise in futility. Nonetheless, calories tally with regards to your weight; this is a reality in which, in science, analyses called overloading studies have been demonstrated on numerous occasions.

These examinations request that people deliberately indulge and, after that, survey the impact on their weight and wellbeing. All overloading investigations have found that people are putting on weight when they devour more calories than they consume.

This simple reality infers that calorie checking and limiting your utilization can be proficient in averting weight put on or weight reduction as long as you can stick to it. One examination found that health improvement plans, including calorie including brought about a typical weight reduction of around 7 lbs. (3.3 kg) more than those that didn't.

Primary concern: You put on weight by eating a bigger number of calories than you consume. Calorie tallying can help you expend fewer calories and get more fit.

How many calories do you have to eat?

What number of calories you need depends on factors such as sex, age, weight, and measure of activity? For example, a 25-year-old male competitor will require a bigger number of calories than a non-practicing 70-year-elderly person. In case you're trying to get in shape, by eating not correctly your body consumes off, you'll have to construct a calorie deficiency. Utilize this adding machine to decide what number of calories you should expend every day (opening in crisp tab). This number cruncher depends on the condition of Mifflin-St Jeor, an exact method to evaluate calorie prerequisites.

How to Reduce your Caloric Intake for Weight Loss

Bit sizes have risen, and a solitary dinner may give twofold or triple what the regular individual needs in a sitting at certain cafés. "Segment mutilation" is the term used to depict huge parts of sustenance as the standard. It might bring about weight put on and weight reduction. In general, people don't evaluate the amount they spend. Tallying calories can help you battle indulging by giving you a more grounded information of the amount you expend.

In any case, you have to record portions of sustenance appropriately for it to work. Here are a couple of well-known strategies for estimating segment sizes: Scales: Weighing your sustenance is the required approach to decide the amount you eat. This might be tedious, in any case, and isn't always down to earth.

Estimating cups: Standard estimations of amount are, to some degree, quicker and less complex to use than a scale, yet can some of the time be tedious and unbalanced.

Examinations: It's quick and easy to utilize correlations with popular items, especially in case you're away from home. It's considerably less exact, however.

Contrasted with family unit items, here are some mainstream serving sizes that gauge your serving sizes:

1 serving of rice or pasta

(1/2 a cup): a PC mouse or adjusted bunch.

1 Meat serving (3 oz): a card deck.

1 Fish serving (3 oz): visit book.

1 Cheese serving (1.5 oz): a lipstick or thumb size.

1 Fresh organic product serving (1/2 cup): a tennis ball.

1 Green verdant vegetable serving (1 cup): baseball.

1 Vegetable serving (1/2 cup): a mouse PC.

1 Olive oil teaspoon: 1 fingertip.

2 Peanut margarine tablespoons: a ping pong ball.

Calorie tallying, notwithstanding when gauging and estimating partitions, isn't an exact science.

In any case, your estimations shouldn't be thoroughly spot-on. Simply guarantee that your utilization is recorded as effectively as would be prudent. You should be mindful of marking high-fat and sugar things, for example, pizza, dessert, and oils. Under-recording these meals can make an enormous qualification between your genuine and recorded utilization. You can endeavor to utilize scales toward the beginning to give you an excellent idea of what a segment resembles to upgrade your evaluations. This should help you to be increasingly exact, even after you quit utilizing them.

More Tips to Assist in Caloric Control

Here are five more calorie tallying tips:

• Get prepared: get a calorie counting application or web device before you start, choose how to evaluate or gauge parcels, and make a feast plan.

• Read nourishment marks: Food names contain numerous accommodating calories tallying information. Check the recommended segment size on the bundle.

• Remove the allurement: dispose of your home's low-quality nourishment. This will help you select more advantageous bites and make hitting your objectives easier.

• Aim for moderate, steady loss of weight: don't cut too little calories. Even though you will get in shape all the more rapidly, you may feel terrible and be less inclined to adhere to your arrangement.

• Fuel your activity: Diet and exercise are the best health improvement plans. Ensure you devour enough to rehearse your vitality.

Effective Methods for Blasting Calories

To impact calories requires participating in exercises that urge the body to utilize vitality. Aside from checking the calories and guaranteeing you eat the required sum, consuming them is similarly essential for weight reduction. Here, we examine a couple of techniques that can enable you to impact our calories all the more viably.:

1. Indoor cycling: McCall states that around 952 calories for each hour ought to be at 200 watts or higher. On the off chance that the stationary bicycle doesn't demonstrate watts: "this infers you're doing it when your indoor cycling instructor educates you to switch the opposition up!" he proposes.

2. Skiing: around 850 calories for every hour depends on your skiing knowledge. Slow, light exertion won't consume nearly the same number of calories as a lively, fiery effort is going to waste. To challenge yourself and to consume vitality? Attempt to ski tough.

3. Rowing: approximately 816 calories for every hour. The benchmark here is 200 watts; McCall claims it ought to be at a "fiery endeavor." many paddling machines list the showcase watts. Reward: rowing is additionally a stunning back exercise.

4. Jumping rope: about 802 calories for each hour this ought to be at a moderate pace—around 100 skips for each moment—says McCall. Attempt to begin with this bounce rope interim exercise.

5. Kickboxing: approximately 700 calories for every hour. Also, in this class are different sorts of hand to hand fighting, such as Muay Thai with regards to standard boxing, when you are genuine in the ring (a.k.a. Battling another individual), the biggest calorie consumption develops. Be that as it may, many boxing courses additionally incorporate cardio activities, for example, hikers and burpees, so your pulse will in the long run increment more than you would anticipate. What's more, hello, before you can get into the ring, you need to start someplace, isn't that so?

6. Swimming: approximately 680 calories for each hour freestyle works, however as McCall says, you should go for a vivacious 75 yards for each moment. For an easygoing swimmer, this is somewhat forceful. (butterfly stroke is significantly progressively productive if you extravagant it.)

7. Outdoor bicycling: About 680 calories per hour biking at a fast, lively pace will raise your pulse, regardless of whether you are outside or inside. Add to some rocky landscape and mountains and gets significantly more calorie consuming.

The volume of calories devoured is straightforwardly proportionate to the measure of sustenance, just like the kind of nourishment an individual expends. The best way to lessen calories is by being cautious about what you devour and captivating in dynamic physical exercises to consume overabundance calories in your body.

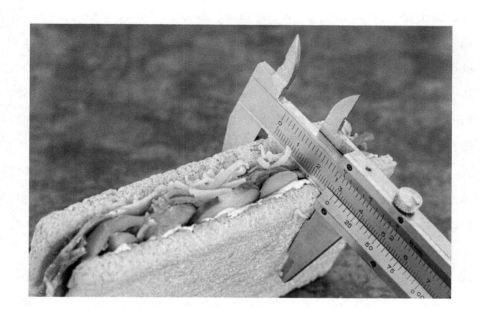

Chapter 10 Lose Weight Fast and Naturally Using Hypnosis

I am going to guide you through different hypnosis now. This one is focused on weight loss. I am going to help you discover the results that you have always wanted, all by unlocking the things in your brain needed to start this process. First, make sure that you are sitting somewhere comfortably. A metronome might help regulate your breathing as well.

Begins by placing your hand on your stomach. As you do this, feel the body that exists underneath. It's not the one you want right now, but it's the one that you have. As you breathe in, feel your stomach expand.

As you let that air out, feel your stomach flatten. Now, count to five with me as you breathe in. One, two, three, four, five. Count to six as you breathe out. Hold for an extra second because I want you to feel your stomach flatten. Become aware of how different your body can change.

Now, sit with your hands somewhere comfortable, focusing only on your closed eyes. Again, keep breathing in and out, noticing the differences that you can feel in your body through your stomach muscles. The things that our bodies are competent to are pretty incredible. Knowing all the abilities we have with them can be very enlightening.

When connected with our bodies and attached to all of the things that they can do, it's going to be much easier to make sure that we are making healthy decisions that are best for them.

Slowly let your mind drift somewhere relaxing. Pick a place in nature. Maybe it's a forest, a beach, or a large grassy field. Wherever it is, I want you to envision this. I'm going to count to ten again, and as I do, your mind is going black.

Now, you see nothing but black. As you focus on nothing, a small light emerges, and you see it starting to grow. As it does, you become more relaxed, still feeling the air enter and exit your body. The light keeps going, and before you know it, it is pouring all over your body.

You suddenly realize that you aren't thinking about this place in nature, you are there. As you look around, there is green surrounding you. The blue sky emerges through the leafy green trees, and you can feel the warm sun start to warm your skin.

A cool breeze comes over your body, and you feel the freshness through your hair. You are not afraid of being alone in this place in nature. It is something that you have been waiting. This is what you deserve.

You start to walk forward, not going anywhere in particular. As you take each step, you begin to see a small building in the distance. You are slowly walking, feeling your body relax. You feel light, fresh, healthy. Something about the way you think now is different than how you did before.

The building is right in front of you now, and you take it upon yourself to walk in. As you open the door, light pours onto you, and you suddenly feel even more rejuvenated. The building is air-conditioned, and you can tell that it is fresh and new. You aren't sure where you are, but it doesn't matter. No one seems to be there, but you are not afraid to be alone. As you walk in, you see a mirror standing right in front of you.

At first, you are afraid to look into it. There might be a person looking back at you that you do not want to see. Something is convincing you that it is time to look into this mirror, however. As you walk up to it, you are shocked to see the person looking back at you. This is a person that you don't recognize at first. They are healthy. They are smiling. Their skin is clear, and their hair is radiant. They are fit, and you can tell that they are working out. The more you look at them, the more you realize that this is you. This is the version that you have been waiting.

You have had visions in the past of what it might look like to decide to go along with your weight loss journey finally. Now, you are here. You are looking into the mirror and seeing a person that you have been hoping for all along. You are happy and healthy. You are confident, and you are excited.

As you look into the mirror, you suddenly remember all that it took to get there. There were moments where you thought that you couldn't do it. There were times when the only thing that felt right was for you to give up. There were many hindrances in your way, but you finally dared to fight through them and get what you wanted.

As you look at your legs, you see that they are strong. They carried you for your entire life, helping you get places that you would never have imagined. You can see the figure of your muscles in them, so strong and sleek. As you move up, you see the flat stomach that you have always wanted.

You might still have a few stretch marks, but they are there to remind you how much you worked for your health. You fought for yourself for your body. You went through things that others aren't able to do on their own. You see this in your torso. All the food that looked so appetizing that you said "no" to shows in your flat stomach now. Every time you chose something healthy instead of something merely tasty is making itself present on your body.

You see that your chest is strong as well. This healthy chest protects your heart, and you can feel it working well as it sends blood throughout your body. You are feeling energized, correct, fulfilled, and happy. Finally, you see your shoulders and arms. These are so strong and have also helped to carry you so far.

You look at them from your fingers to your neck, toned, and supporting the rest of your body. Though you have seen all of the essential changes throughout the rest of your body, the most important thing is how broad your smile is now. Your cheeks are stretched to show the radiance that has always existed inside you and can finally be present.

It feels so good to notice that you look this good, but what is even better than that is that you are so comfortable with your body. Throughout your weight loss, you learned how to take care of yourself in a healthy way so that you will be able to keep the weight off for a long time. There were moments when all you wanted to be a specific body, but right here, smiling into the mirror, you know now that the most important thing is that you are happy.

It is time now for me to bring you out of the hypnosis. When I count to ten, you will be back into the present world, ready to start your journey.

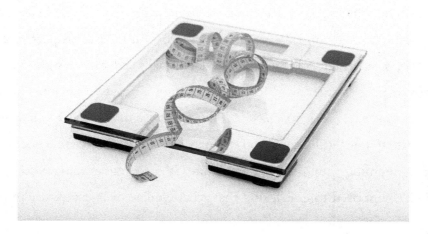

Chapter 11   Hypnotherapy for Weight Loss

You have undoubtedly heard of people who use hypnosis to help them lose weight and how they say it worked for them- just as many others have been helped quit smoking. Yet, do you know how it works?

Weight loss hypnotherapy works when a professional therapist creates a patient's ideal mental environment or action to help achieve a desired outcome or goal. This is when hypnosis can become a collaborator in maintaining weight loss with more traditional methods.

The process of induction usually generates a hypnotic condition. Although there are a variety of weight loss inductions for hypnotherapy, most of them include suggestions for well-being, relaxation, and calm. There are often instructions included in the induction to remind the person or imagine some experiences that were pleasant to them.

It has been shown that everyone reacts differently to hypnosis. Some people will describe hypnosis as just a regular focus of attention while feeling calm and relaxed. It would appear that most hypnotized people found it to be an incredibly pleasant and relaxing experience.

Part of the reason why weight loss hypnotherapy works are that it focuses on what might cause someone to be overweight in the first place. A professional hypnotist's goal is to tap into a subconscious person and reprogram it to alter whatever behavior initially led to the weight gain. Many hypnotists may work on programming a negative response to an action that they want to change. The hypnotist might use a threat like overeating that will cause you to experience sick or hate chocolate, reprogramming your subconscious mind. If the programming works the way it's supposed to, you'll find that when you've over-eaten, you're not feeling perfect or interested in eating candy. Alternatively, by planting the idea that you prefer healthy options for yourself and don't need to consume fattening foods, the hypnotist could choose to reinforce your resolve.

If you consider weight loss hypnotherapy, you might want to check out some of the available self-hypnosis CDs and MP3's. Take a few minutes to check out the weight loss options for hypnotherapy that we would like to suggest.

Several people have been found to have a strong response to suggestions given under hypnosis, while others are not as successful reactive. Often fears of an individual may hinder their ability to integrate the hypnotic suggestions given to them, usually based on misconceptions. When someone is hypnotized, they are still aware of what is going on and control their actions, as opposed to how it is depicted in books, television, or movies. We are usually mindful of themselves and their surroundings, and unless otherwise mentioned, they are knowledgeable and remember whatever happens while being hypnotized. Hypnosis is meant to encourage people's acceptance of ideas, but it never goes against their will or pressures them to embrace unwelcome changes.

For treating pain, anxiety, depression, bad habits, stress, and many other medical and psychological issues, several people have found help with hypnosis.

If you're serious about trying weight loss hypnotherapy, there are quite a few excellent therapists online and self-hypnosis tapes and books with which you can operate independently.

With the exponential rise in the number of people struggling to meet their ideal weight loss targets, there has arisen another possible method of tackling overweight. Hypnotherapy is reliable, results-oriented, and non-invasive for weight loss. One of the main reasons for its popularity is that the treatment does not require consulting doctors, buying vitamins, undertaking intense physical exercises, or even going on a low-carbohydrate diet, etc. The weight watcher can do hypnotherapy for weight loss-at most he or she can seek assistance from a professional hypnotist. However, many can study and practice hypnotherapy at home through various tools of self-help available.

Weight loss hypnotherapy isn't the only place where hypnosis is used. It is one of the most promising treatment methods for treating various mental and physical conditions, including pain control, depression, anxiety attacks, addictions, and much more. The therapy method's effectiveness is corroborated by the fact that even doctors now recommend hypnotherapy for permanent weight loss and refer licensed hypnotizers to their overweight patients.

The weight loss can be achieved in two ways by hypnosis. The first approach is to see a qualified hypnotist, who will lead you through the hypnotism process. However, for others, the cost of care using a hypnotist's services can be an obstacle. You can take the second choice in these cases, which is self-hypnosis. There's no better help than self-help, after all.

Self-hypnosis is not a daunting activity, and there are numerous self-help devices such as MP3 hypnosis, etc., which can be used in the comfort of your home to learn and practice the art. You don't have to hit the gym or buy those pricey diet pills to shed those extra pounds. Weight loss hypnotherapy has proven successful, and there's no reason why it shouldn't deliver the desired result for you too.

Hypnosis works to lose weight because it operates at the subconscious level of the mind, the layer from which most of our cravings, phobias, fears, and apprehensions arise. Hypnosis gets to the root of the overeating problem, lack of motivation to do physical activities, cravings for unhealthy foods, etc. by first soothing the mind and then inserting various constructive ideas that the peaceful mind picks upon. Hypnotherapy for weight loss is so effective because it changes the outlook on food. You become a more rational person, capable of separating the good and the bad. You are turned into a more optimistic individual who sets and succeeds in achieving practical weight loss goals.

Can something as easy as weight loss hypnotherapy be the solution you've been searching for in your fight to drop the pounds and hold the fat away forever? Having a hypnotherapist is becoming increasingly common these days for all sorts of health problems such as giving up smoking, overcoming phobias, and being thinner successfully.

How does hypnotherapy work to help someone lose weight?

Being able to come off the street and get hypnotherapy done on you is not normal. You usually have to make an appointment first (and sometimes multiple follow-ups, too).

The hypnotherapist will ask you a series of questions, then start putting you into a trance.

The trance has three phases to it. The first step is induction, which is close to the counting down often that you may have seen on television before. The second is a deepening level; as the deeper you are in a trance, the more open you are to suggestions you will be. There's the awakening point, at last.

Why is it successful?

You are given a series of powerful suggestions during a hypnosis session. These stay with you when you return to reality but may lose their influence over time.

This is why having multiple sessions to reinforce the desired results is relatively standard. The success rate is relatively poor, with only one session.

The hypnotherapist's ability also has a major impact on how effective it can be. Better ones will tailor their sessions precisely to you and not just regurgitate the same scripts they are using for all their other clients. This is because you might find the reasons for your weight issue special, and so only tailor-made solutions can work well for you.

The evidence on how practical this approach is very scarce and can not be believed to be unbiased by the own data of explicit hypnotherapists. Roughly half of those who take hypnosis can expect some form of weight loss success from it with repeat sessions.

How can I obtain access to it?

Hypnotherapists are found throughout the world. The critical thing to remember is that medical practitioners are not approved. Nevertheless, you might be able to access it through the national health service or insurance plan.

However, most people would have to pay for those programs. Look for qualified accreditations and testimonials from past clients while finding a successful hypnotherapist to give your money.

You can also listen to digital audio files, which are also a modern way of self-hypnosis if you don't have access to a local specialist. But don't expect quite the same success levels anywhere compared to using a licensed hypnotherapist's services.

Chapter 12   What is Self-Hypnosis?

Self-hypnosis is still considered a mystical phenomenon by many people, even though this technique can be seen as prayer. You are alone, and you concentrate on your well-being. If you like, you ask God or a supreme being you believe in to help you. This practice includes meditation (just like praying does) and chanting, mantras, inner confirmation or affirmation. When you have to perform at work or college, you make such statements like "I don't fear; I'm fine"; "I can do it" or precisely the opposite, like "I can't do it. Everybody is better than me," etc. Even when we imagine ourselves in a different scenario from what is currently happening, we are programming ourselves. What you are doing is continuously hypnotizing yourself. Self-hypnosis helps us come into contact with the unconscious through the use of a specific language, aimed at awakening some parts of ourselves by leveraging archetypal symbols. Self-hypnotization is self-programming. Our unconscious understands the symbolic messages of words rather than their rational meaning; that's why figurative language is used in hypnosis to induce the individual to relax and focus on the inner world. We are embedding a vivid, information-rich image with emotions in the subconscious mind.

However, we must learn to pray, or let's say hypnotize ourselves accurately! Self-hypnosis is the ability to apply techniques and procedures alone to stimulate the unconscious to become our ally and involve it directly in realizing our goals. By learning the essential elements of communication with the unconscious mind, it is possible to reprogram our unconscious activities. Self-hypnosis is a method that does not dismiss the support of a professional but has the advantage of being able to be performed independently. This is possible through the use of CDs and DIY courses made by hypnotists to make this practice accessible to a larger number of people with significant advantages, even from an economic point of view!

What is self-hypnosis?

Milton H. Erickson, the founder of modern hypnotherapy, gave an exhaustive illustration of the effects and purposes of hypnosis and self-hypnosis. The scholar stated that this practice aims to communicate with the subconscious of the subjects through metaphors and stories full of symbolic meanings (Tyrrell, 2014).

If incorrectly applied, self-hypnosis can certainly not harm, but it may not be useful in attaining the desired results, with the risk of not feeling motivated to continue a constructive relationship with the unconscious. However, to do it as efficiently as possible, we need to be in a relaxed state of mind. So, accordingly, we start with relaxation to gather the attention inside, while suspending conscious control. Then we insert suggestions and affirmations to the unconscious mind. At the end of the period allocated for the process, a gradual awakening procedure facilitates returning to permanent consciousness. When you are calm, your subconscious is 20-25% more programmable than when you are agitated. Also, it effectively relieves stress (you can repair a lot of information and stimuli you understand), aids regeneration, energizes, triggers positive physiological changes, improves concentration, helps you find solutions, and helps you make the right decisions. If the state of conscious trance is reached, if the patient manages to let himself go by concentrating on the hypnotist's words, progressively forgetting the external stimuli, the physiological parameters undergo considerable variations. The confirmation comes from science. It was found that during hypnosis, the left hemisphere, the rational one, decreases its activity in favor of the more creative region, the right one (Harris, n. d.).

You can do self-hypnosis in faster and more immediate ways, even during the various daily activities after experiencing what state you need to reach during hypnosis.

A better understanding of communication with the unconscious mind highlights how indispensable our collaboration is to slip into the state outside the ordinary consciousness. In other words, we enter an altered state of consciousness because we want it, and every form of hypnosis, even if induced by someone else, is always self-hypnosis.

We wish to access the extraordinary power of unconscious creativity; for this, we understand that it is necessary to put aside the control of the rational mind and let ourselves slip entirely into relaxation and the magical world of the unconscious.

Immense benefits can be obtained from a relationship that becomes natural and habitual with one's unconscious. Self-hypnosis favors the emergence of constructive responses from our being, allows us to know ourselves better, helps us be more aware of our potential, and can express them and use them to foster our success in every field of possible application.

How do you do self-hypnosis?

There are several self-hypnosis techniques out there; however, they are all based on one concept: focusing on a single idea, object, image, or word. This is the key that opens the door to trance. You can achieve focus in many ways, so there are so many different techniques that can be applied. After a period of initial learning, those who have learned a method, and have continued to practice it, realize that they can skip specific steps. We will take a look at the essential self-hypnosis techniques.

The Betty Erickson Method

Here I'll summarize the most practical points of this method of Betty Erickson, wife of Milton Erickson, the most famous hypnotist of 1900.

Choose something you don't like about yourself. Turn it into an image, and then turn this image into a positive one. If you don't want your body shape, take a picture of your body, then turn it into a copy of your beautiful self with a body you would like to have. Before inducing self-hypnosis, give yourself a time limit before hypnotizing yourself mentally or better yet, saying aloud the following sentence, "I induce self-hypnosis for X minutes." Your mind will take time like a Swiss watch.

How do you practice?

Take three objects around you, preferably small and bright, like a door handle, a light spot on a painting, etc. and fix your attention. Take three sounds from your environment, traffic, fridge noise, etc., and set your attention on each one. Take three sensations you are feeling, the itchy nose, tingling in the leg, the feeling of air passing through the nose, etc. It's better to use unusual sensations, such as the sensation of the right foot inside the shoe, to which attention is not usually drawn. Don't fix your attention for too long, just enough to make you aware of what you are seeing, feeling, or trying. The mind is quick. Then, in the same way, switch to two objects, two sounds, two sensations. Always be calm, while switching to an object, a sound, a feeling. If you have done things properly, you are in a trance, ready for the next step.

Now let your mind wander, as you did in class when the teacher spoke and you looked out of the window, and you were in another place, in another time, in another space, in a place where you would have liked to be, so completely forget about everything else. Now recall the initial image. Perhaps the mind wanders, from time to time it gets distracted, maybe it goes adrift, but it doesn't matter. As soon as you can, take the initial image, and start working on it. Do not make efforts to try to remind you of what it means or what it is. Your mind works according to mental associations, let it work at its best without unnecessarily disturbing it: it knows what it must do. Manipulate the image, play with it a little. See if it looks brighter, or if it is smaller, or it is more pleasant. If it is a moving image, send it back and forth in slow motion or speed it up. When the initial image always gets worse, replace it instantly with the second image.

Reorientation, also known as awakening, marks the end of self-hypnotic induction. Enjoy your new image, savor it as much as you like, and open your eyes when you have done this. If you have not given yourself any time limits before entering self-hypnosis, when you are satisfied with the work done, count quietly to yourself from one to ten and wake up, and open your eyes (Traversa, 2018).

The Benson Method

Herbert Benson, in his famous book titled, Relaxation Response, describes the methods and results of some tests carried out on a group of meditators dedicated to "transcendental meditation" to reach concentration (1975). Benson suggested a way of relaxation based on the mind's frequency on a single idea incorporated in the Eastern disciplines. The technique includes the following steps:

● Meditate on one word, but you can choose an object or something else if you want to.

● Think silently about the object of meditation and continue to do so for 10-20 minutes. If you find that you have lost the object of meditation, gather your focus again on the original purpose.

● Once the set time is reached, open your eyes stretch yourself well for some additional minutes. To perform better, you will need to practice.

Benson proposes this exercise as a meditation practice. There are no differences between the hypnotic state and that achieved with meditation. This is one of the most straightforward self-hypnosis exercises you can do.

Here is another simple technique developed by the first hypnotists because it leads to a satisfactory state of trance in a reasonable time. It can be used to enter self-hypnosis in a short time.

● Begin to open and close your eyes by counting slowly. Open your eyes at the odd numbers close them at the even numbers. Continue counting very slowly and slowing down the numbering of even numbers.

● After a few numbers, your eyes become tired, and you find it difficult to open them at odd numbers. Continue counting while you can open your eyes at the different names. If you cannot do it, it means you are in a trance.

● Go deeper by slowly counting twenty other numbers. Let yourself go to the images, sensations, and the words that come to mind. To wake up from the trance, count from one to five, and open your eyes at five (Stress Management Plus, n. d.).

These are examples of techniques, but no one prevents you from devising others, as long as the underlying assumption is maintained: concentration on a single idea.

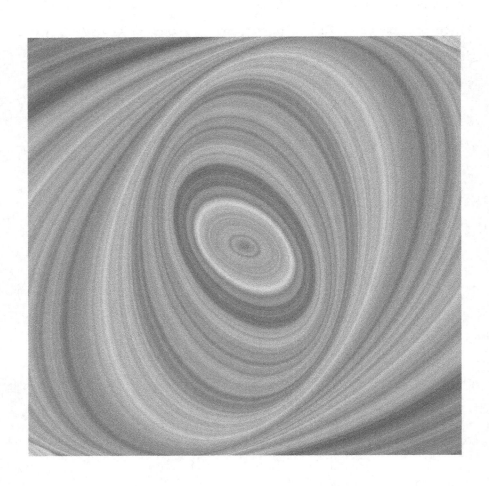

Chapter 13   Practicing Hypnosis Techniques

We all need time to relax, to dream, to pretend. It is clean to the bodily frame and rejuvenating to the spirit. When we practice our hypnosis, it offers us just that: a completely personal time to liven up and increase our thoughts and frame. The exercise is done. You need nothing extra than a cushy and safe place.

A Few Simple Rules

There are some guidelines to hypnosis, and they make sure that your practice is the most efficient and yields the finest benefits. When you're prepared to begin the usage of the audio, locate a cushy and safe place in your own home or workplace in which you can sit in a chair, recline, or even lie down. Make sure you're comfortable and in a place where you no longer have to be aware of something else. Do not listen to your trance work simultaneously as you're using an automobile or running any machinery. It is useful to decide on an ordinary time each day or night time to exercise your self-hypnosis. Bedtime is a superb possibility to experience your trance work, and practicing at this time can be a great way to go into a restful sleep.

Distractions and interruptions are inevitable. Rather than allowing them to bother you and take you far from your trance work, use them. Use the sounds inside the surroundings around you to beautify your trance enjoy. For instance, even as doing your hypnosis, you may note a valid and start questioning that this sound is distracting you. You then turn out to be more focused on this distraction than for your hypnosis. You may be tempted to struggle in opposition to it—which takes electricity away from the hypnosis instead, while you be aware of a sound that before everything seems distracting or traumatic, take control of it using giving it your permission to be there as a background sound. Give it an assignment, such as questioning yourself that "the sound of the barking dog is helping me cross deeper and deeper within" or "the fan motor appears like a waterfall that is a soothing history sound." At our exercise in Tucson, there is a day college that necessarily shall we the children out to play for the duration of one in every of our hypnosis sessions. When we recommend, "The sound of children may be a background sound that helps you pass deeper and deeper within yourself now." This is a part of our "use everything" philosophy.

Distractions also consist of the sensations you might enjoy inside you. For instance, you could discover yourself noticing part of your body that itches. The closer your attention to the itching or on scratching the itch, the less you focus your cognizance on the trance. At the one's times, you indeed remind yourself that you have permission to transport your attention back to your trance or daydream and let the itch go unscratched. When working with patients who've pain disorders, we educate them to concentration far from the "distraction" of ache in a similar manner.

After all, we cannot manage the surroundings round us or the sensations inside us; however, we can pick out in which we awareness our interest. If you have a problem letting move of an annoying distraction, you may command that or not it's there as a history sound or sensation, which then makes you go higher with ease inside. Detach yourself from something that is competing along with your interest in your hypnosis. Let pass any warfare with the environment. Just allow it to be there, and sooner or later, you will now not be aware of it. When you discover ways to take delivery of a sensation, noise, or other elements that interferes with your hypnosis, you now not allow it to have to manage over you.

Law of Reversed Effect

There is a regulation in hypnosis, referred to as the Law of Reversed Effect, that asserts that occasionally the greater you try to do something, the more it does now not happen. An instance is while you need to say a call which you realize you understand—it can be a book title, a person, a movie—however, you cannot say it at that moment, and the more you try, the less it's far there. The call comes while you advise your subconscious mind that "I'll take into account later" or "It'll come to me later." By letting cross of the question, "What's the name? What's the name?" you have launched your subconscious mind to now retrieve and supply the answer, and it usually does. So, the Law of Reversed Effect is that while you are attempting too tricky for something, it most effective gives you the opposite (the reverse).

Simple Techniques

Becoming absorbed in your thoughts and ideas is that gentle adventure into the middle of yourself known as "going into a trance." The simple self-hypnosis strategies encompass going into a trance, deepening the trance, using that trance state to provide messages and guidelines to the thoughts-body, and coming out of a trance.

Meanwhile, do recognize that the subconscious mind (or unconscious mind) is the part of our psyche that performs functions and techniques under our thinking focus. It is the thoughts of the frame. It breathes us, digests, pulses our hearts, and in general, manages our involuntary physical procedures for us. It can also inform us to pick out a piece of clean mango instead of chocolate cake, to stop eating while we're full, or to experience a walk in the park.

Also, the conscious mind is the "thinking mind" or the part of the psyche that gives us our cognizance or experience of understanding and governs our optional features. For example, our conscious mind takes that 2nd piece of pie at the buffet, swipes the debit card at the grocery store, and actions the fork to our mouth.

Going into Trance

When you use the trancework on the audio, I could be your manual as you move into a trance. I will use a trance induction technique that you may find calming and focusing. You have likely seen the swinging watch approach in movies, which is thirty-five years of practice I have in no way visible all people use, but there are many different ways to cognizance your attention to enter a trance. You might stare at a gap on the wall, use a respiration technique, or use innovative body relaxation.

You will pay attention to a variety of induction methods at the trance paintings audio. They are simply the cues or the signals that you are giving to yourself to say, "I am going into a trance" or "I am going to do my hypnosis now." Going into a trance can also be the concept of as "letting your self-daydream ... Deliberately." You are letting yourself grow to be absorbed in your thoughts and thoughts, very incorporated, and permitting yourself to pretend or believe what your preference as performed and real. There is no "going under." Instead, there may be a lovely revel in of going within.

Deepening the Trance

Deepening your trance allows you to end up extra absorbed in your thoughts, thoughts, and enjoy. This is accomplished with innovative relaxation: going "deeper and deeper inside." with pics or scenes, or counting a number sequence. We like to signify that as you listen to counting from ten down to zero, you create vertical imagery related to going deeper, along with a direct main down a mountain or into a lush green valley. As you pay attention to me counting, you could picture or imagine going more deeply right into a scene or place. This is even extra enjoyable and snug to you. This is what we suggest via "deepening the trance."

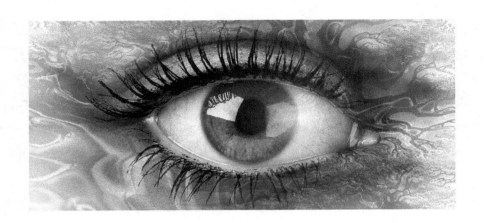

Chapter 14   How much does it Cost for Weight Loss Hypnosis?

Exactly how can we validate the price distinction between the signed-up Stomach Mind Band ® Permanent Weight Loss Treatment and the many other Hypnosis centers providing what seems a comparable therapy, at often half the cost? We comprehend that some people, for a range of reasons, are concentrated purely on the value of their treatment, leading them to find for the most affordable weight-loss hypnosis type clinic they can find, and additionally question why to take a trip to Spain if you can finish the therapy closer to the residence.

Nevertheless, you need to recognize that high quality and obtaining permanent weight-loss results are identified with a cost. For instance, the rate for hypnotherapy for weight loss kind treatment in the UK, whether you are seeking to stop smoking cigarettes or reduce weight ranges between £ 125 to £ 475 per session, typically lasts for an hour. However, when it involves the critical location of your long-term wellness, we believe making a dedication, and your financial investment should be the driving factor in your choice, together with investigating that you entrust to aid you in this essential location your life. In the future, selecting a hypnotherapist or hypnosis facility with experience as well as the best certifications to back them up together with tested as well as released outcomes will undoubtedly give you with the worth as well as with any luck, the results you desire, require as well as naturally, are worthy.

You should additionally be mindful that the study has shown that Hypnotherapy as a stand-alone method hardly ever provides long-term leads to the weight management field. As defined on the many web pages of the GMB site, our therapy is based around several proven Psychological interventions, underpinned with Hypnotherapy, which is hugely different, as well as the result of over 10 years of research and development at the Elite Weight Loss Clinic.

The chart listed below displays what we provide. Besides basic hypnotherapy, allow us to guarantee you, you will undoubtedly experience a lot greater than just sitting in a chair relaxing. Your wellness is our very first priority, along with providing irreversible fat burning results. As you will see below, we require as well as apply complete health and wellness evaluation, which includes full blood and body analysis tests.

The main point is if you're searching for inexpensive hypnosis after that, you're most likely to discover much less worth. We've created a graph showing you how various we are, not just as a result of our years of experience, accreditations, as well as education. Yet, additionally, due to the value, we supply to our clients. We provide a Gold Basic solution, including full Skype or Face Time follow-ups, we provide complete assist before and after our treatment and walk with you every action of the means on your weight reduction journey.

We need you to do your research and look for other hypnotherapy centers using weight-loss therapy and specific hypnotherapists. Learn what they supply for the rate entailed than simply compare it with our graph below. Lastly, perhaps ask yourself why over a thousand people, both stars and participants of the general public, have circumnavigated the globe to experience the GMB Therapy in Spain.

Treatment Components GMB-- Elite Spain Others

· Minimum of 16 hrs of one to one therapy time, solely with Martin and also Marion Shirran. Red Enigma

· Therapy includes full, professional blood examinations and analysis. Including overall Cholesterol, HDL as well as LDL Cholesterol, Triglycerides, short term fasting Glucose (blood glucose) as well as Hemoglobin A1c (HbA1c), which gives your average blood sugar level degrees over the previous three months. Red Question Mark

· Complete Tanita Body evaluation examinations were taken on, consisting of fat mass, body fat percentage, and also visceral overweight rating. The test likewise confirms your unique 'Metabolic Finger Print.' Red Enigma

· Treatment includes four sessions of CBT, PBT, Clinical Hypnosis, and also NLP. Red Enigma

· Committed session around the current innovative Nutritional Info, confirmed to be crucial for attaining long-term weight loss. Red Question Mark

· Medical Proof of therapy efficiency, as offered at International Psychology Conferences published on the facility's website. Red Enigma

· Distinct Forensic Weight Reduction Survey ® established in-house, utilized to make sure that each client is dealt with as a person. Red Enigma

· All customers are dealt with mainly by the GMB developers as well as authors. Red Question Mark

· Each session is electronically videotaped, making it possible for clients to duplicate components at home. Red Enigma

· Pulse Oximeter (Heart Monitor) used during Medical Hypnotherapy sessions to guarantee the right degree and deepness of relaxation. Red Question Mark

· Full 50-page GMB workbook/manual offered to every client following their therapy. Red Question Mark

· Over 1,000 clients already treated unedited and also verified case studies and pictures released. Red Enigma

· Regular follows up Skype/ FaceTime sessions complying with therapy conclusion. The therapy will not stop, no matter if you leave the center. Red Enigma

· Establish of weight-loss devices unique to GMB treatment and presented per customer. Red Question Mark

· Independent Media reviews of GMB Treatment, both Press and TV, published on the facility website. Red Enigma

· Treatment is embarked on at the specialized clever, contemporary, and fully furnished Elite Clinic, located in Southern Spain, merely twenty mins from Malaga airport. Red Enigma

· Each client presented with authorized copies of the writer's books, as released around the world by Hay Home. Red Enigma

· GMB therapy subject to continual and also on-going Research and Development.

Hypnotherapy is commonly used for weight management, smoking cessation, stress and anxiety, anxieties, laziness, low self-worth, insomnia, sexual performance problems, and various other issues.

Common expenses

Hypnosis sometimes is covered by health insurance. However, it differs by plan and individual instance. For example, BlueCross BlueShield of

Montana thinks about hypnosis that is clinically necessary for alleviating intense or persistent discomfort or as a complement to psychotherapy. Aetna, nonetheless, takes into consideration hypnosis experimental. For patients covered by medical insurance, the price of hypnosis usually includes a doctor browse through copay or coinsurance of 10%-50%.

For individuals not covered by medical insurance, hypnotherapy generally sets you back $50-$275 or more per session-- or a total of $100-$1,375 or even more for both to five sessions typically advised for the majority of problems. For example, Columbus Ohio Hypnosis bills $50-$100 per session, depending on the carrier, with three to 5 sessions typically called for, for an overall of $150-$500. Possibilities Hypnotherapy Centers in Massachusetts and Rhode Island charge $95 per session and also suggest two sessions for smoking cigarettes and even 3 for fat burning-- for a total amount of $190-$285. Shore Counseling & Hypnosis Center in North Carolina charges $110 per session-- with up to three or more sessions advised, for an overall of up to $330 or more. Brennan Smith, a hypnotherapist in California, bills $145 per session, with 3 to 8 sessions recommended, for a total of $435-$1,160. Absolute Peak Hypnotherapy Center in Ohio bills $275 per session, and also needs two sessions to stop cigarette smoking and even 3 to 5 sessions to reduce weight, for a total of $550-$1,375.

If you're thinking of utilizing hypnotherapy to deal with a problem, you may be asking yourself, how much does hypnosis cost? One size does not fit all. Or in the case of hypnotherapy, one rate does not fit all. The cost of hypnosis is different and fluctuates from city to city-- from one acupuncturist to the following.

In this article, we'll explore the costs you can anticipate when you look for hypnotherapy treatment, the kinds of discount rates you may be qualified for, how to locate affordable hypnosis, and hypnotherapy costs in several of the major cities.

If you're thinking about spending for hypnotherapy therapy via insurance coverage, we'll reveal which insurance provider will certainly spend for hypnotherapy therapy, as well as if you're seeking a particular treatment for smoking, or weight loss, we'll likewise offer you an idea of what you can anticipate spending for those treatments.

Fees for your first session of hypnotherapy might consist of a first consultation as well as hypnotherapy therapy. This will cost between $100 to $300. Additional goals might cost $75 to $300. Some hypnotherapists supply a free 30-minute first in-person or phone consultation to get a feeling if you are comfortable dealing with the hypnotherapist and to aide in discovering the hypnotherapist for both your wellness and health demands.

Price cuts

Many acupuncturists provide a discount rate when you acquire numerous treatments or plans. For example, if you were to get one session at $150 or six sessions at $600, bringing the cost down to $100 per session.

· Other popular discount rates are:

· Reference discount rates

· Review discount rates

· Student Price cuts

· Kid Discounts

· Senior discounts

· Expert Discounts

· Teacher discounts

Ask your hypnotherapist if they provide any one of these discounts to obtain a better treatment rate.

Overall Price

The total cost of hypnotherapy will depend on the kind and also factor you are seeking hypnotherapy. Individuals have spent greater than $300 out of pocket throughout their full treatment for hypnotherapy. Some people have spent $500 or even more. Nevertheless, do not worry; hypnotherapy does not have to be financially unreachable.

Exactly How to Find Inexpensive Hypnotherapy

Along with asking hypnotherapists if they supply any type of discounts, one other means to locate affordable hypnotherapy treatment is to ask a hypnotherapist if they provide a sliding range cost timetable. It is a fantastic method to make hypnosis a much more budget-friendly therapy alternative for your health requirements.

When a hypnotherapist gets their certification or is dealing with obtaining their certification, they are often needed to complete a specific variety of hypnotherapy hours.

One other avenue of finding low-cost hypnotherapy sessions is locating a hypnotherapist who is to find a hypnotherapist who is functioning in the direction of meeting those needed hours of hypnosis for their accreditation well as aiming to construct their hypnosis organizations. Since they are starting, they might agree to supply a reduced hypnosis session per hour rate to expand their customer base and the company.

Which Insurance Companies Cover Hypnotherapy?

The complying with insurance companies might cover your hypnotherapy, depending upon your strategy. Be sure to get in contact with your insurance coverage supplier to validate coverage before looking for therapy. Your hypnotherapist might also have the ability to assist you.

· Blue Shield: Will cover hypnotherapy for chronic discomfort and if it is done in addition to psychotherapy relying on the strategy you have.

· Cigna: Will certainly cover hypnosis if hypnosis is being utilized to deal with a protected condition and also depends on the strategy you are spending.

· Humana: Honestly, blog sites about hypnosis and anxiety.

· United Health Care: Various plans might cover hypnotherapy for analysis or therapeutic objectives.

The insurer Aetna thinks about hypnotherapy and hypnotherapy as experimental and investigates and, consequently, will not cover it.

Chapter 15   Is Meditation the Same as Self Hypnosis?

Many people confuse one of these terms with the other, and authors tend to make this problem worse by using them interchangeably in their writing. Meditation and Self-hypnosis are relaxing and a very effective way to reduce stress and calm the mind and body. However, there are crucial differences. Let's take a closer look at these two related but different relaxation methods.

What is Meditation?

Meditation is a relaxation method to calm the mind. It can be achieved by focusing on something specific. It can be your breath, an object, or a particular phrase or word. When you meditate with open eyes, you generally focus on an object in the room. On the other hand, if you meditate with your eyes closed, you are more likely to focus on breathing or repeating a specific phrase or word. This is called "mantra," and it is usually repeated either silently or out loud.

Focusing on something specific is an essential feature of meditation; therefore, when thoughts arise, you will notice them briefly. Once you do, you want to quickly and carefully return your attention to the center of your meditation practice.

The Aim of Meditation

Meditation aims to calm your mind and make you feel calmer. This will help you feel happier and relax. It enables you to be more present, and it's also great to improve concentration by focusing on one thing. You will notice more of your thoughts and feelings with improved self-awareness.

Meditation helps you reach a calm state of mind or perhaps an altered state of consciousness. It happens when beta brain waves (our normal active brain state) go to the alpha level: meditation is often part of a broader spiritual practice.

Meditation may or may not be guided. Guided meditation requires listening to a recording (or a person). Become your center of focus. The voice then guides you to focus on different things. It can be your breath, different parts of your body, or positive words and phrases. You can also add guided imagery to help you relax with your imagination.

With unguided meditation, you do it yourself, focusing on your breathing, an object, or a mantra. You focus on one thing and notice what your mind is doing. And you can meditate almost anywhere!

In my opinion, guided meditations are very similar to self-hypnosis recordings. Either way, focus your mind on the content of the record. With guided meditations, the purpose of the suggestions is to help you achieve a calmer mind. A self-hypnosis recording can also do this, but it will often focus on changing a habit, behavior, or experience of something you want to happen in your imagination.

Guided meditation can also help you reprogram your subconscious as well as self-hypnosis recording. Both reach the relaxed state necessary to consider positive ideas and suggestions at a deeper level.

What is Self-Hypnosis?

Hypnosis can be done by another person, such as a hypnotherapist or hypnotist. However, self-hypnosis is when you hypnotize yourself. Hypnosis's general purpose is to bypass your conscious mind, access your subconscious, and make changes unconscious.

With a self-hypnosis recording, you listen to another person and are guided through a hypnotic technique or process. Hypnosis, therefore, includes access to the subconscious. That is why we use various methods to achieve positive changes.

The Aim of Hypnosis

Self-hypnosis often involves the use of positive suggestions. When you are relaxed, tips, positive ideas, or affirmations reach a much deeper level in your subconscious mind. Self-hypnosis is very useful in dealing with and changing feelings, experiences, resolving fears, accessing resources, controlling obstacles, habits, and emotions. It is often challenging to locate a rational, conscious waking state. Self-hypnosis is commonly used to eliminate or reduce physical pain and discomfort.

Similarities Between Meditation and Self-Hypnosis

Both involve achieving an altered state of consciousness, with beta brain waves moving to the slowest alpha level.

The two have to do with a kind of dissociation. Be less aware of your physical environment and the external world and develop more internal attention. This makes you more aware of your feelings, thoughts, and emotions.

Both involve focused attention or concentration. For meditation, this can be your breath, an object, a mantra, or a recording. For self-hypnosis, these would be the suggestions from the hypnotherapist or a record of self-hypnosis.

The Difference Between Meditation and Self-Hypnosis

It looks like a straightforward question, but when you take a closer look, you see that there are so many various techniques in the two categories that make it difficult to do more than a general comparison. Although the boundary between meditation and self-hypnosis is not clearly defined, I think it is possible to distinguish it.

Hypnosis, whether self-hypnosis or administered by someone else, is actively trying to reach a part of your mind for a specific purpose. For example, if it is part of a therapy session, hypnosis can be used to explore hidden or repressed memories of the subconscious and draw the user's attention. It allows the person to overcome the problems. Hypnosis can also be used to create a positive state of mind by repeatedly citing key phrases called "affirmative statements." They can help make subconscious changes by continually putting the thought into your conscious mind and waiting for it to seep through the subconscious, which is the root of the problem and the key to the solutions.

Hypnotherapy generally points to a more specific outcome. It can be weight loss, quitting smoking, phobia elimination, etc. At the beginning of a hypnotherapy session, meditation techniques can calm the conscious part of the mind. Once the chattering consciousness is silent, it can provide the subconscious mind with agreed therapeutic suggestions. Therefore, the recommendation seeks a specific therapeutic objective. Hypnotherapy focuses on a particular therapeutic outcome.

Meditation is designed to help you focus your mind and center it on nothing. Yes, I said nothing because it is the most challenging thing for our conscious mind to do. Outside of periods of sleep or unconsciousness, our waking moments are filled with thoughts that we are unaware. When you sit down and try to clear yourself, do you realize how difficult it can be? It would help if you had specific techniques to achieve this state of mind where you don't consciously think about something in particular.

Traditional meditation is generally less structured. Meditation is often described as the absence of all thoughts. In meditation, you strive to maintain a state of calmness without consciously chattering. When conscious thoughts arise in words during meditation, you need to find a way to get rid of them. Meditating is at peace with who you are and what you do.

Meeting the expectations of others or even our expectations of ourselves causes stress. However, meditation can free your mind from all these negative thoughts and feelings and make you experience inner peace. In meditation, we want to have a calm mind, free from conscious thoughts.

A hypnosis session and a meditation session can lead you to a state of deep relaxation and guided visualization on a tranquil and calm beach. However, a hypnosis session will use this state of mind to suggest a therapeutic change in the subconscious mind. A person who meditates benefits from the tranquility and relaxation he experiences. This peace of mind can lead to enlightenment and self-improvement by improving the overall mind.

Hypnosis and meditation can cause deep relaxation. The two can claim a host of similar health benefits, but the pathways to the same destination are slightly different. In this sense, self-hypnosis is active, while meditation is passive. With self-hypnosis, you create change, while with meditation, you allow making adjustments by getting out of the way. Both are very effective for personal transformation but in very different ways. Both are relatively simple and easy to learn.

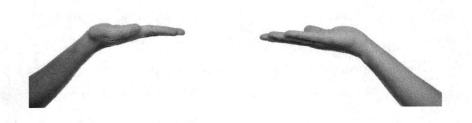

Chapter 16   What is Meditation?

To many people, the technique appears somewhat vague and difficult to grasp without giving it a bit of time to see the results. To some, the battle with the fleeting mind only discourages them from taking a step further to calm the mind. To others, religious dogma stands in their way. Some folks have chosen to embrace the practice and report numerous benefits, some even taking up journeys to go and meditate in every known meditation center. It is entirely okay to belong to any of these groups because it requires a lot of dedication and open-mindedness, without which the method may appear dull or unfruitful. It is a practice for a reason!

Yet, what is this phenomenon called "meditation"? Meditation is a practice that involves the application of various techniques such as breathing and mindfulness to achieve a calm mental state and train focus and attention. The primary purpose of the practice is to help you observe your feelings and emotions without judgment with the benefit that you will get to understand them well. Therefore, meditation does not make you a holy person or a different person, but it has the potential to if you wish to take the path.

What is not meditation? Meditation is not a practice meant to make you high or zone out or even have bizarre experiences. Many people carry this notion around with them. It would be good to eliminate some of these thoughts before getting yourself to start the practice lest you feel deceived. Meditation is an avenue to train your mind in awareness.

History of Meditation

Whether you are new to the concept or are already a guru about reaching enlightenment, learning about this practice's history is very important. Wall art in India that shows people seated in the meditation pose with closed eyes appeared approximately 5,000 to 3,500 BC serve as one of the oldest documented proof of the practice. Even so, the oldest written records of the practice trace back to the Vedas in 1,500 BC. Nevertheless, for them to write it down, the practice passed down orally for over centuries.

Anciently, meditation was a practice of the religious and practitioners of asceticism. These people abandoned all the pleasures of the world to transcend themselves over life's limitations.

Around the 6th Century BC, the Buddha Siddhartha Gautama, a prince at the time, decided to abandon the palace and find enlightenment. He disposed himself to the best yogis he could find in his region but was still unsatisfied with his results. He decided to go into the forest, sit under a tree, and meditate until he achieved what he direly craved. He was fruitful enough to discover his technique of meditation and achieve enlightenment. He spent the rest of his life serving people and teaching them this practice. The spread of Buddhism ensued over the next centuries, and its lineages are some of the most famous modes of meditation in the West.

Confucianism, Taoism, and Jainism received birth in the same Century that Buddha existed but have their approach towards the meditation practice. Confucianism focusses more on morality, Taoism with universal life, and Jainism on self-discipline, non-violence, and purification of the self. Although still practiced today, they do not much enjoy Yoga and Buddhism outside of their home countries.

The cultural influence propagated by Alexander the Great's military activities from 327 to 325 BC brought Indians and Greek philosophers in touch. Under the control of yogis and sages, the Greek philosophers were able to form their version of meditation-navel gazing. Popularly known as omphaloskepsis, philosophers' common practice was to assist them in their philosophical thoughts. This meditation technique did not hold for so long as other philosophers such as Plotinus and Philo of Alexandria developed different methods that dealt with concentration. Moreover, the Christian crusades that dominated the West eventually snuffed out these traditions until later on in the 20th Century.

Mystics from the Christian pool also developed their form of meditation. Its characteristics were the contemplation of God and repetitions of individual words or phrases that held divine meaning. A popular way of meditation is the Jesus Prayer, which sprouted in Greece between the 10th and 14th Century. According to historian speculations, their influence of meditation occurred when a group of Christians ran into the Indians and the Sufis. Benedictine monks are responsible for the further development of Christian meditation.

While visiting China, Dosho, a Japanese monk, discovered Zen's art and introduced the practice into his country when he returned. He also opened the first meditation hall. The method gained popularity in the 8th Century with Japan, Korea, and Vietnam adopting the practice.

The mystics of Islam, popularly known as the Sufis, introduced meditation that revolved around gazing, mantras, and breathing. They received some of their influence from Indian traditions. The primary purpose of their meditation practice is to have a connection with God. In Turkey today, the Sufi swirl (also developed by them) is still noticeable.

Meditation continued to develop and grow during the Middle Ages as religious traditions masked in forms of prayers like the Jewish meditation. Meditation teachings saw their popularity amid Western cultures during this time. Meditation has been able to traverse many narrow pathways and reach the ears of many since then.

Science was able to tap into the resource of meditation in the 1930s. James Funderburk, a student of the Himalayan Institute of Yoga Science, made studies of scientific research on meditation possible in 1977. He was a student of Swami Rama, one of the first yogis studied by scientists from the West. Under scientific observation in the '60s, Swami Rama displayed his ability to control his blood pressure voluntarily, body temperature, and heartbeat. Among other things, he also displaced the ability to:

- Produce delta, alpha, gamma, and theta brain waves on-demand.
- Remain environmentally conscious while still in a deep sleep.
- Manipulate his heartbeat while assuming a motionless pose and stopping his heart for a couple of seconds.
- Generate different skin temperatures on different sides of his hand.

This led to the popularization of scientific studies on meditation over the next five decades. As the quality of machines increased, the quality of these findings also increased. However, meditation (during this time) was highly referred to as a religious practice, some of these feats set in motion the end of this belief. Meditation is a form of healthcare, thanks to this.

Presently, the practice of meditation is experiencing secular and mainstream recognition, mostly to influence wellness of mind and body. This does not mean that spiritual meditation has seen its end. The practice is still in motion. However, it is the value of wellness that still acts as the most significant attraction to meditation practice.

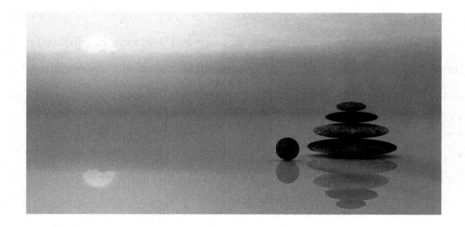

Chapter 17   Guided Meditation for Weight Loss

Reducing extra pounds is the problem, perhaps, of every woman who requires a lot of work, courage, patience, and willpower. But often the hours spent on the simulator, strenuous exercises, exhausting hunger strikes do not give the desired result; weight loss does not occur. But many people do not even realize that you can lose weight using a simple and enjoyable way. This slimming meditation is a simple and natural tool that will help promote progress in weight loss.

Meditation is often seen as a relaxing practice, but it benefits the mind only, not the body. When you think "I have to lose weight," you will tend to see yourself exercising more and dieting. However, the first step in these two methods is going through your head. So we will see how we can effectively practice meditation to lose weight.

How Meditation Helps Lose Weight

It would seem that how meditation can help women lose weight? But in fact, meditation practice has many advantages:

- Metabolism regulation. With regular exercise, the human body restores its biological functions, including metabolism. This contributes to the fact that weight loss occurs naturally, fat deposits go away. A proper metabolism in the body also causes a decrease in appetite, which is why a person eats less.

- Digestion. Meditation helps to improve the absorption of food. Hormonal imbalances in the female body and stress lead to overeating and indigestion. Regular exercise helps relax your nerves and balance hormones. This has a long-term impact on efforts to reduce extra pounds.

- Legibleness in food. One of the hindrances to weight loss is the craving for unhealthy and unhealthy foods. Slimming meditation eliminates these unhealthy urges. A person becomes more attentive to what he eats, as he takes care of his own body and therefore loses weight.
- Stress resistance. Very often, overeating occurs due to stress. Experiencing, a person himself does not notice the growth of his appetite. This leads to a set of extra pounds. That is why meditation is essential for losing weight because it eliminates the primary source of the problem and reduces stress.
- Discipline. Uncontrolled meals and snacks are associated with the fact that a person can not refuse his favorite food. The only way to perfection is faith in oneself, willpower, clarity of mind, and discipline. By meditating regularly, all these qualities can be developed and strengthened in oneself.
- Self-hypnosis. Much is known about the power of thought - they materialize and become a reality if efforts are made. In this case, meditation works like hypnosis - a person programs himself for the result.

How to lose weight while meditating

Meditation on harmony should be a daily practice. For effectiveness, it is recommended to meditate daily for at least 20 minutes.

Slimming meditation does not have to be complicated. If you're a beginner, try starting five minutes in the morning to clear your mind before confronting a busy day and five minutes before going to bed.

Yoga instructors note that, in principle, the time of classes does not matter if you meditate regularly and correctly.

The rules of meditation if you want to lose weight:

- Use a mantra to help you lose weight. A mantra is a phrase that you will repeat to yourself to focus on the goal when your mind wanders. These are words that can eventually enter into meditative hypnosis.

- Watch your breath. Just close your eyes and focus on your breath without trying to change it. If your mind wanders — and it will be so at first — just direct it back to your breath.

- Meditation for excellence in losing weight should not be stressful. In the process, a person should feel comfortable, which applies to everything: clothing, posture, environment, and well-being.

- Step-by-step instruction

- Anyone who wants to lose weight can meditate. There is no need for expensive classes. For many, the hardest part is simply looking for the time. But on the road to your goal, you can do it.

- Make sure you have the opportunity to create silence for the time you need.

- When you find yourself in a quiet place, calm yourself, relax. You can sit or lie down in whichever convenient position.

- Start by focusing on your breath, observing your chest or stomach when it rises and falls. Feel the air as it moves and exits your mouth or nose. Listen to the sounds that the atmosphere makes. Do this for a 1-2 minutes until you begin to feel more relaxed.

- Then, with your eyes open or closed, do the following: Take a deep breath. Hold it for a few seconds. Exhale slowly and repeat. Inhale naturally. Observe your breathing when it enters your nostrils, raise your chest, or move your stomach, but do not alter it. Keep focusing your breath for 5-10 minutes.
- Start to visualize. Imagine how slim and beautiful you put on your favorite dress, how you walk along the catwalk, and how men turn around. In weight loss meditation, women need to increase their self-esteem and understand that change is necessary for their perfection.

Meditation Results for Weight Loss

If you want to meditate correctly to lose weight, look for exercises focused on this. Losing weight meditation looks more like hypnosis or self-hypnosis. It is essential to form the power of thought, the power of will. It is necessary to impress yourself that you want something (to lose weight in this situation) and strive to fulfill your desire.

This can be a visualization of how you can look and feel after you have lost weight. You can imagine yourself slim and thin, mentally put on your favorite clothes.

But with all the benefits of meditation when losing weight, it is only one method in a set of actions for losing weight. It is impossible to lose weight, just meditating. If you eat kilograms of chips and buns and can not reduce your appetite, then even many hours of meditation will not save you and will not help to reduce weight.

Proper nutrition and exercise are also essential parts of the path to harmony. There will always be better results if you combine all these components into one and make them your way of life.

First of all, meditative practice changes the thinking, consciousness, and attitude to the problem, strengthening desire and desire. Studies show that these changes take only 21 days. It is in three weeks that a person's habits change and form, including eating right and eating little, refusing junk food, and drinking plenty of water - this also helps to lose weight.

As you can see, meditation is the key to harmony, an amazing technique in which there is no single side effect. This practice can change a person, both internally and physically, for the better.

Benefits of Meditation for Weight Loss

1. Get more energy.

Meditating for three to five minutes a day gives your mind and body a chance to rest, relax, rejuvenate, and refresh your body to every cell.

2. Feel Good.

The better you feel, the more comfortable you'll be to lose the pounds. Instead of grabbing a sweet cake, try meditating for a few minutes until the craving goes away. Try that!

3. Better focus.

The more you meditate, the more you can concentrate. Meditation is also a practice in which specific thoughts are based. The more you can focus, the more you can focus on meeting your weight goals.

4. Reduce Stress and Anxiety.

Some individuals go to the gym to relieve tension, and meditation may take place. Even if you exorcize the body and still have tension, the body still retains all this tension. If the mind holds you back, the body will hold you back. Why not both. Why not.

5. Lose Weight.

The physiology of the body is usually such that what we do, sound and think affects the energy and sensations in each cell of each organ of our body. Meditation is one of the easiest ways to control the body and lose weight.

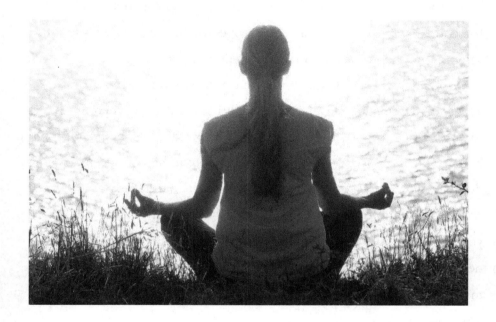

Chapter 18   Fat Burning Meditation

This fat-burning meditation is a simple 30-minute meditation that allows you to visualize your fat cells, reducing into smaller and smaller cells until they virtually vanish. Focusing on these types of hypnosis, meditations are said to help direct your subconscious mind to interact with your body so that you can begin to have a healthier and healthier body. When you focus on intentionally drawing your subconscious awareness into these activities, it encourages it to continue engaging in these activities on its own, even when you are not involved in your hypnosis session.

This is a great meditation to engage in during the day anywhere from one to three times per week, or at bedtime. They say that meditating right before you fall asleep can be particularly potent, as you are meditating during a time where your subconscious mind is particularly active. Your conscious mind is already beginning to fall asleep. Throughout this time, you are most likely to experience the level of relaxation and receptivity needed for your subconscious mind to digest the changes you seek to make within it.

The Meditation

To begin this meditation, allow yourself to close your eyes and start to fade into a deep state of relaxation. Feel yourself relaxing and deeper with each breath, and notice yourself falling into a beautiful state of calmness. To help you deepen your relaxation, I will guide you through a practice that will take you to the deepest level of relaxation. To do this, I want you to visualize yourself standing at the top of a set of stairs. As I count down from 10 to 1, I want you to imagine yourself walking down that flight of stairs, taking just one step. With each step you take, visualize yourself relaxing deeper and deeper until you find yourself in a deep state of relaxation and ready to engage in a hypnotic visualization session.

Beginning with ten, visualize yourself taking a step down the stairs. Notice your surroundings, including the color of the walls, what the bottom step looks like, and any decorations surrounding you. With nine, step down again, and see yourself getting closer to the bottom of the flight of stairs. Notice your relaxation doubling with every step you take, as you step down to the eighth step. Notice how your perspective may be changing around you as you descend lower and lower down the stairs, moving down to the seventh stair. Now, step down to the sixth stair. When you are ready, step again down to the fifth stair, feeling your relaxation doubling once again as you sink deeper into a state of relaxation and calm. Now, step down to the fourth stair. As you look before you, you can see a chair coming into your view when you step down again to the third stair. As you step down to the second stair, you can see that the chair looks incredibly comfy, and you cannot wait to feel your relaxation triple when you sit in it as you step down to the first stair and then off the stairs.

When you get off the stairs at the bottom, see yourself walking up to that chair and sitting in it. Notice that this chair is the comfiest chair you have ever sat in, and upon sitting in it, you feel your entire state relaxing ten times deeper as you sink into the chair. Feel yourself becoming so calm that you can fade away in this space.

As you sit there, notice your awareness turning inward into your body. As your knowledge turns inward, draw your focus down into your fat cells. See each cell sitting there, hugging your body, and keeping you warm and

117

comfortable in your current state. Notice how each cell feels confident that it serves a purpose, and sits proudly in its position. As you look at each of these fat cells, realize that they are not there to cause you harm or destruction, but because they genuinely believe they are meant to be there. They think they are serving an essential job for you and your life.

As you draw your awareness even closer into these cells, I want you to pick one up in your hand. See this small round cell sitting in your hand, proudly serving a purpose in your life. As you hold it, thank the cell for all that it has done, and with complete gratitude, let it know that you no longer need it to help you anymore. Cup the cell between your hands and feel it shrinking down until it vanishes between your palms.

Again, pick up another cell and hold it in your hands. With sincere gratitude in your heart, thank it for serving its purpose and let it know that you no longer need its help. Wish it well as you cup it between your palms and shrink it down until it vanishes.

Keep doing this with your fat cells as you continue to pick them up, express gratitude for their service, and then shrink them down in your palms until they vanish entirely. One by one, let each fat cell know that it is no longer needed and that you are grateful for all that it has provided you with until this point in your life. Let your remaining cells know that you now require less fat to restore your health and start to feel better and better.

As you get to the end of the fat cells, notice that you look around and no fat cells remain. All you see are healthy cells that support essential functions in your body like cell regrowth, digestion, and circulation. Express sincere gratitude for every single cell in your body and its work, and allow yourself to release this perspective as you draw your awareness

118

back into your body. See your awareness growing beyond the size of your small cells and back into the knowledge of yourself as you come back into the room where you presently sit. Feel yourself awakening from your meditation now, as you open your eyes and feel different within your body.

From now on, when you go through your daily life, notice how even though some of your fat cells continue to remain, you can almost see them disappearing. Continue to express gratitude for each cell and all that it has done to attempt to support your survival, and allow it to peacefully fade away as you allow yourself to come back into a state of lean health.

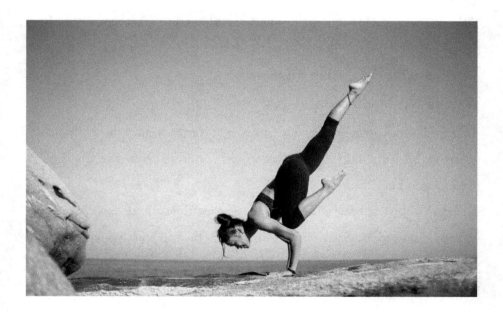

Chapter 19 Meditation for a More Energized Morning

Sometimes, a part of waking up is doing so in a relaxed way. You might have to chill out a little bit before you will be able to wake yourself up fully!

If we go too fast all day, it can feel like we never fully get a break. This meditation is great for those who have a bit of extra time in the morning to relax for a minute before heading off. It can also be great for those who might want to listen to something as they eat breakfast, drink their morning coffee, or stay in bed for a few moments longer while becoming more energized.

This one was not designed to put you to sleep, but since it will still be a relaxing reading, you will want to ensure that you are in a safe location on the chance that you do drift off to sleep.

Waking Up Meditation

A new day has just begun, and now, it is time to start fresh. You are going to be launching a brand new with nothing from the day before holding you back.

To begin your day off right, it is time to relax. Relaxing doesn't mean that you are going to be tired. This means that you will start your day with a clear head, a calm body, and a rested soul.

For this, you will want to do an exercise in which you make a fist, sticking your pinky and thumb out with your right hand. Now, place your right pinky on your left nostril, pressing down. Now, breathe in through your right nose. Then, take your right thumb and press on your right nostril, lifting your pinky. Then release your air through your left nostril.

The point of this is to alternate the nostrils in which you breathe in and breathe out. You will start to see how this can quickly calm you down.

Do this again as we count. Breathe in for one, two, three, four, and five. Breathe out for six, seven, eight, nine, and ten.

Once more, breathe in for ten, nine, eight, seven, six, and out for five, four, three, two, and one. Repeat the breathing exercise throughout the day when you need to calm down. Whenever you start to feel the panic rise at any time, try out this great exercise. It helps you focus on something while also ensuring that you are regulating your breathing.

Now, it is time to close your eyes and focus on becoming refreshed and new. You are going to start this day off right without anyone else distracting you. There aren't going to be things that keep you down. You are centered only on feeling as good as possible, all the time.

We are lucky to have a brand-new day each day. Although we might have to do the same things as we did the day before, it is time that we look at these things with a fresh mind. We can start over.

Release yourself from what happened before this moment. Remain proud of your accomplishments, but forgive yourself for some of the decisions that you might have made. Keep your memories around, but only for proper use. Remember the great times and learn from your mistakes. Don't ruminate on thoughts.

Prepare yourself to confront what you might need to face today. Remember that you are healthy and powerful, someone who is capable of absolutely anything. You can do all the things that you have dreamed of being able to do. No matter what you place in your mind, the results that you want will come.

Embrace the new day. Let yourself be open to what others might bring today as well. How will the people you know be different from yesterday? Can you forgive others and mistakes that they might have made?

Breathe in positive vibes. Breathe out the fear that you have today.

Breathe in new experiences, breathe out your anxiety over what these experiences might bring.

Accept that even the things that might be challenging for you will also bring you new knowledge. Even things that seem scary or out of reach will give you new experiences you never thought possible. You will go through things beyond anything that you could easily imagine. You will always be tested on your strength, willpower, and resilience.

Take everything with pride. Assure yourself that you are capable of anything. Remember how brave you can be. Nothing is going to keep you afraid today. There are no things that you might confront that will bring you fear.

Breathe in the bravery that you need to conquer this day. Breathe out all of the feelings that you might not be able to do it. Remember how far you have come already.

You are not going to repeat what happened yesterday, or the day before, or the day before. Even if you did something great today, you would do even better.

You are going to make healthy choices throughout the day to help you feel like your best self. You will provide your body with nutrients, energy, and everything else it needs to function as well as possible.

Remember to stay relaxed and stress-free throughout the day. When you free yourself from stress, you are letting go of all the things that might be holding you back. When you say "no" to anxiety, then you are granting yourself the chance to be happy and content with what you have and with the things that currently surround you.

You are letting yourself go from the things that have held you back in the past. Your eyes are open now, and you see all that is needed to do to have the best day possible.

You are awake, alert, and energized. You are centered on breathing healthily and living happily.

You are not afraid of what is to come. You are entirely well-rested and have had all of the sleep that you need to be happy throughout the day.

You have the chance to go to sleep later. You will have the ability to start over once again then tomorrow. No one can stop you from reaching greatness today.

As a final way to wake up, we are going to do one last quick hypnotic exercise. You are awake and alert now, but this will help you feel even more energized to have the best day possible. Every day will be the best day because you will learn how to show gratitude, grow, and be entirely content.

Right now, continue to focus on your breathing. Keep your eyes open and hold your hand up so that you can snap it on command. With your eyes open, look up as high as you can without moving your head. This will result in your vision being slightly cut off by your eyelids.

Look up as high as you can using your eyes only, but not to the point that you are straining or hurting them. When we count down from three, snap your fingers on one and look in front of you. This will help quickly kick you awake and give you a little jolt of energy.

Keep looking up, higher and higher. On one, snap your fingers and look straight ahead. Three… Two…. One….

You are now awake, energized, and ready for the day.

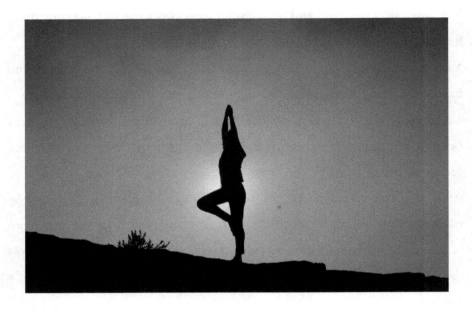

Chapter 20   Hypnotic Gastric Band

What Is a Gastric Band?

A gastric band is a silicone device that is commonly used to treat obesity.

The device is usually placed on the upper part of the stomach to decrease the amount of food you eat. While on the upper part of the stomach, the band makes a relatively smaller pouch that fills up quickly and slows the consumption rate.

The band works when you make healthy food options, reduce appetite, and limit food intake and volume.

However, it leaves you with a difficult option of bariatric surgery, a drastic step that carries the usual risks and pains like any other gastrointestinal surgical operation. You do not need to experience these challenges when there is a simple and less invasive approach to achieve the same results as in a surgical gastric band.

Hypnotic Gastric Band

If you would like to lose some weight without having to involve surgery, then the hypnotic gastric band is the tool you need.

It is a natural healthy eating tool that can help control your appetite and your portion sizes. In this sense, hypnosis plays a significant role in helping you lose weight without the risk that comes with surgery.

It is a subconscious suggestion that you already have a gastric band to influence the body to respond by creating a feeling of satiety.

It is now in the public domain that dieting does not solve lifestyle challenges required for weight loss and management.

Temporary diet plans are less effective, while continuous plans are challenging to maintain. Notably, these plans deprive you of your favorite foods and are too restrictive.

Deep down, you may have a problem with your body weight, and perhaps diets have not worked for you so far.

If you wish to try something that will provide a positive edge, you need to control your cravings around food hypnotically. By reaching this point, it is clear that you are prepared to try hypnosis, which has proven to aid weight loss.

How Does Hypnotic Gastric Band Work?

Typically, the conscious mind is not as receptive to suggestions, for it frequently analyzes and critiques it.

You empower the mind to accept suggestions in a deep and relaxed state. This way, you can reframe your thinking patterns due to the principles of disassociation and opinion. With the hypnotic gastric band, you use suggestions to influence a different response from the body triggered by sensory data to create a new reality. The proposals provide a guideline that you are supposed to follow without questioning or critiquing. Ultimately, this power enables you to reframe and reshape your perception regarding a specific behavior.

Chiefly, the complex network in your brain has different interpretations of the world around you, and most probably unhelpful and negative thoughts may have worked their way into that network.

As a result, you automatically become susceptible to uncontrolled unconscious urges such us overeating and ignoring serious bodyweight concerns. The hypnotic gastric band helps you dampen and overcome these uncontrolled thoughts and believe in suggestions that play a significant role in altering your behavior.

Powerful affirmations: A change in lifestyle is mandatory if you wish to have permanent weight loss or control. Powerful affirmations are vital in changing your lifestyle slowly and surely.

Therefore, you should diligently practice regular affirmations for weight loss to realize the dream of losing weight. Notably, weight control is a direct function of your lifestyle as you are solely responsible for your behavior. Your mental attitude determines your weight, the rest you take, physical exertion, and manner and frequency of eating. Use effective weight loss affirmations as a way to initiate the measure from your mind.

For real, it is necessary to change your thinking; otherwise, no form of dieting will ever help. Weight loss affirmations are significant in your mind, making you feel the comfort in your desired weight.

You should also consider the affirmations' wording to ensure that you focus on the solution but not the problem. For instance, you should not say, "I am not that fat," for that is the problem. Instead, you must focus on the solution and include words such as "I am getting slimmer" or "I am losing weight daily."

Write down healthy weight affirmations or take a cue from the samples I will provide. Repeating them shows that you are determined and sure to take the bold step of living and looking at a fitter life.

I weigh _ pounds: This affirmation sets the desired weight in your mind, and as you repeat the words, you remind yourself about your destiny and measures that you need to take.

I will achieve the ideal weight to enhance my physical fitness: You embrace lighter weight and improve physical activity.

I love healthy food, for they help me attain an ideal weight: It promotes healthy eating and craving for healthy food.

I ease digestion by chewing all the food properly to reach my ideal weight: The affirmation is perfect before every meal as it guides the rate and amount of consumption.

I control my weight through a combination of healthy eating and controlling my appetite and my portion sizes:

It is good to repeat these affirmations, among others, especially in front of a mirror, to remind your subconscious mind about your goals. Most importantly, these affirmations work best while meditating or in a trance state. This combination will do wonders in your weight loss endeavor.

Powerful Visualization: With a hypnotic gastric band, your imagination should control your subconscious mind and body.

Visualizing weight loss means making the image of how you want to be in your mind's eye. It is a wonderful tool that triggers the subconscious mind to shape your body to match your mental image. If you visualize accordingly, you will achieve weight loss, improve how you look, and become more energetic. Notably, emotions and thoughts affect the body for better or for worse. Negative thinking, anger, fear, stress, and worry, hurt the body and lead to the production of toxins that adversely affect you. If you are happy, confident, and positive, you energize and strengthen the body.

Learning how to use your subconscious mind in visualization effectively is to your advantage. Besides, it is a mental diet that you should incorporate in your weight loss plan. Chiefly, the success of the hypnotic gastric band will be higher if you eat healthily in addition to affirmations and visualization.

Visualization is such a vital tool in the journey of leaving overeating and emotional eating behind. The significance of display lies not in our physical body but in the feeling of overcoming obsessions and challenges with food, weight, perfect body or plagues, and restrictions that keep you on the dieting merry go round.

With the hypnotic gastric band, visualization is a simple process, and you can use these few tips for weight loss.

- Find frequent moments where you sit down for several minutes and quietly visualize your slim body. Ignore all doubts, worries, and negative thoughts and maintain focus on the image.

- Forget your current look and imagine a beautiful and slim you with the ideal weight. See how gorgeous you look in a swimming suit and tight clothing that you always want to wear.

- Visualize peers and family complimenting your slim body and looks. Just watch the whole scene as if it is real and happening now.

- Feel free to construct different versions of these instances or other physical roles, such as dancing or swimming. Visualize yourself hearing compliments from other people about your slim body and watch them admiringly glare at you.

- Make the images you make in your mind colorful, realistic, and alive. See yourself in each of these real and exciting scenes in the ideal weight.

Avoid words that may destroy the efforts you may have made and let only the thoughts of your ideal weight and shape into your mind. Powerful visualization works wonders when practiced in hypnosis, for it makes the mental image a possible reality.

Why Is Hypnotic Gastric Band Recommendable?

If you would like to lose weight without starvation or yo-yo dieting, then the hypnotic gastric band is the ultimate resort. This gastric band does not require surgery but only meditation and hypnosis. Therefore, it offers numerous benefits that make it the solution to rapid weight loss and craving healthy food.

It is pain-free: As opposed to the physical gastric band, the hypnotic gastric band does not require surgery associated with pain and routine follow-ups. Therefore, you don't have to worry about the risks you need to take, as no physical operation will be done on your body. You only need to hypnotize and utilize the hypnosis to work on your body weight.

100% safe: As hypnosis is a non-invasive, non-surgical, and safe technique, so is the hypnotic gastric band whose mechanism is initiated in your subconscious mind. Through the practice, there are no expected dangers, and you learn about self-awareness and the course of your life.

Time-efficient: You do not need to wait for your vacation to acquire a hypnotic gastric band. The tool does not affect your schedule as hypnosis can be combined with most of your day to day activities. You do not need time off to adjust the band or report complications

No meal replacement or dieting: With the hypnotic gastric band, you do not need to stop eating your most enjoyable food. Instead, you develop a principle that makes you feel in control and enable you to lose weight

130

consistently and naturally without dieting. You exercise and unlock the power in you to make positive changes in life.

No complications: No surgery is performed in hypnotic gastric surgery puts away the worry about future complications. The ease in your mind plays a significant role in focusing your mind on the things that matter, such as visualization and meditation. This way, you can put off negative thinking and live your life fearlessly and positively.

Helps discover your hidden potential: The use of hypnosis and meditation makes you learn how to use your mind's power to change your perception and erase negative thoughts. Similarly, you become capable of helping not only with weight loss but also with other psychological and social aspects such as confidence. Hypnosis helps plant a subconscious suggestion in your mind making it stick and become a strong idea.

Cost-Effective: Hypnotic gastric band does not snatch away your working time, making you fully productive at your workplace with no deductions. In the same way, there are no costs in hypnosis and meditation than the physical gastric band. Positively living your life adds to your savings.

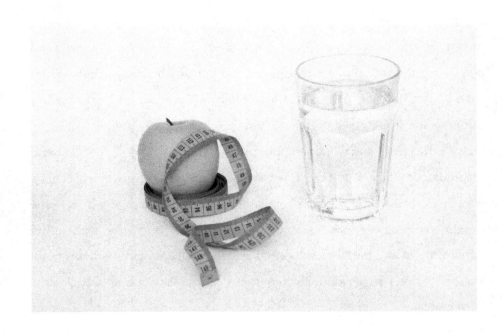

Chapter 21   Hypnotic Gastric Virtual Band

What is the virtual gastric band?

The virtual gastric band is a technique that combines hypnosis and subliminal reprogramming to make the stomach believe that it is smaller than it is to reduce food intake and promote weight loss.

This form of treatment is based on the belief that obesity is a permanent problem. The patient has to learn to eat a balanced diet voluntarily and effortlessly to avoid the rebound effect. Through hypnosis, the patient receives messages of healthy routines that he will put into practice after the session.

Virtual gastric band procedure

This technique acts similarly to those of stomach reduction, limits the amount of food ingested to lose weight. To get the feeling of satiety without using any external device, the patient must attend a hypnosis session. When the patient is semi-unconscious, he will receive subliminal messages to decrease the desire to eat and adopt new healthier eating routines.

This procedure, based on psychological techniques of cognitive-behavioral therapy (CBT) to change habits, must be reinforced from time to time. The messages are losing strength over time, especially in long treatments. Also, to receive recordings that the patient will hear periodically, he must attend other hypnosis sessions to adapt the messages according to the moment he is.

This technique acts like other stomach reduction procedures such as the gastric band, hence its name. The patient will take less food as the stomach will send the satiety message to the brain before it is filled. The virtual gastric band can also be a complementary technique to other surgical treatments or not for stomach reduction, helping the patient acquire the new routines without much effort.

Advantages and disadvantages

The main advantage of a virtual gastric band treatment is that there is no surgical intervention of any kind; it is non-invasive. Therefore, it does not require hospitalization, nor does it leave scars even if they are minimal.

In general, the cost of a virtual gastric band treatment is usually lower than that of other stomach reduction techniques.

However, virtual gastric band treatment is a relatively new technique for which there is not enough scientific evidence of long-term results.

The patient must also have some implications because he must attend reinforcement sessions so that the subliminal messages do not lose strength. Weight gain in obese people is a long-term treatment.

Lose Weight with the Gastric Virtual Band

How many times have you considered losing weight? And how many others have you made a diet that you have abandoned because of the effort involved in getting rid of those extra pounds?

Have you ever raised that the causes are not only biological, that there must be psychological, emotional, or unconscious causes that make you continue to eat disproportionately or compulsively?

Ask yourself if you want to lose weight, and if so, we can propose a new, revolutionary and effective method, it is the gastric virtual band with hypnosis.

A painless, risk-free, and secure method, as we provide it to you.

What is the virtual gastric band by the hypnosis method?

As you have read in the initial questions, and undoubtedly the answers have been often referred to as the first approach and concerning the second one, I am sure you have also thought about it once. Still, you do not find a connection, that is, how you could imagine that it is not that you eat for eating. Again, you often eat for anxiety, frustration, disappointment, boredom, comfort you, etc. You eat your emotions.

At this last point, clinical hypnosis does its job since many behavior patterns, especially those related to food, are learned and automatic.

Through clinical hypnosis, we access the subconscious and create a series of suggestions to recreate an operation of a virtual gastric band that will allow the person to eat and notice satiety as if they had operated on you, but without the side effects that may occur. Produce a real operation, since many people do not know how to identify the limit of their satiety physically.

Therefore, by implanting the gastric band through clinical hypnosis, the brain acts in the same way as if it were inserted since the mind believes it.

In the same way, we make a series of suggestions for each person to start eating naturally, without forcing anything, in a healthy and balanced way knowing when to stop and control, for example, when eating chocolate that does not eat all the box.

On the other hand, and through another series of suggestions or hypnotic programming, we make the person reduce or eliminate the desire that drives him to eat. Usually, the food he usually eats has many calories or sugar that later become fat. It is in extra kilos.

On the other hand, we create hypnotic suggestions to motivate people to move their bodies in any way, walking, exercising, but in such a way that these activities are carried out by people without that mental and physical effort that often involves them.

In some people, if necessary, we could find out through regressive clinical hypnosis if the causes of your overweight are related to some trauma or are the product of a child's behavior that you continue to perform as compensation or refuge from what is affecting you and not solve.

In short, both through the implantation of the virtual gastric band by hypnosis and by issuing specific suggestions for each patient, we can get people to eliminate those kilos more definitively since at the end of the treatment we teach them a self-hypnosis technique so that they reinforce their new beliefs that emit so much with food, their figure thus achieving maintenance over time.

How does Virtual Gastric Band Work

A virtual gastric band is presented as an alternative to diet slim. But how does it work? Each session consists of four sessions of 20 minutes each and follows four primary guidelines. The goal is to stop thinking about food all the time. It's simple in theory, but it can be a bit more challenging to do it logically. For simplicity, this method includes self-help advice, materials, and daily audio. In the second session, the stomach band is placed by hypnosis. There is no type of surgery, but due to hypnosis (does not cause pain or imply any health risks or side effects), the subconscious believes that the stomach has a stomach band and behaves as if it were Smaller). Therefore, you can eat less, feel fuller faster, and lose the kilos you need to reach your ideal weight.

Remember that food is often used for anxiety, boredom, or indifference. In this way, you eat from hunger, not from stress. This means that virtual stomach bands and mental control will save you kilos and adopt healthier eating habits. One of the goals of a slim diet is to retrain your practices when you eat.

The virtual gastric band method is specially designed for those who want to lose a few pounds more and are overweight or obese. Also, people who can no longer lose weight while on a diet, or when food is a substitute for anxiety. It is not recommended for eating disorders (anorexia or bulimia), diabetes, or irritable bowel syndrome.

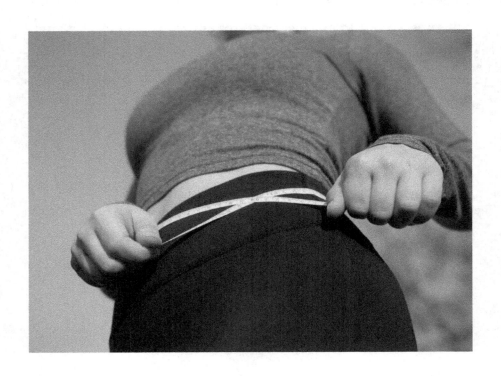

Chapter 22   Preparing   your   Body   for   your
Hypnotic Gastric Band

The physical gastric band requires a surgical procedure that involves reducing the size of your stomach pocket to accommodate less volume of food. As a result of the stretching of the stomach walls, send signals to the brain that you are filled and therefore need to stop eating any further.

The hypnotic gastric band also works in the same manner, although, in this case, the only surgical tools you will need are your mind and your body, and the significant part is, you can conduct the procedure yourself. The hypnotic gastric band also conditions your mind and body to restrict excess consumption of food after very modest meals. There are three specific differences between the surgical (physical), and hypnotic gastric bands:

- In using the hypnotic band, all necessary adjustments are made by the continued use of trance.
- There is an absence of physical surgery, and therefore, you are exposed to no risks at all.
- When compared with the surgical gastric band, the hypnotic gastric band is cheaper and easier to do.

How Hypnosis Improves Communication between Stomach and Brain

How would you know when you have had enough to eat? Initially, you will begin to feel the weight and area of the food. When your stomach is full, the food presses against and extends the stomach well, and the nerve endings in the walls of the stomach respond. When these nerves are stimulated, they transfer a signal to the brain, and we get the feeling of satiety.

 And, as the stomach fills up and food enters the digestive tract, PYY and GLP-1 is released and trigger a feeling of satiety in the brain that additionally prompts us to quit eating.

Sadly, when individuals always overeat, they become desensitized to both the nerve signals and the neuropeptide signaling system. During the initial installation trance, we use hypnotic and images to re-sensitize the brain to these signs. Your hypnotic band restores the full effect of these nervous and neuropeptide messages. With the benefits of hypnotic in view, we can recalibrate this system and increase your sensitivity to these signs, so you feel full and truly satisfied when you have eaten enough to fill that little pouch at the top of your stomach.

A hypnotic gastric band causes your body to carry on precisely as if you have carried out surgical operation. It contracts your stomach and adjusts the signals from your stomach to your brain, so you feel full rapidly. The hypnotic band uses a few unique attributes of hypnotic. As a matter of first importance, hypnotic permits us to talk to parts of the body and mind that are not under conscious control. Interestingly as it might appear, in a trance, we can convince the body to carry on distinctively even though our conscious mind has no methods for coordinating that change.

The Power of The Gastric Band

A renowned and dramatic case of hypnotic power to influence our bodies directly is in the emergency treatment of burns. A few doctors have used hypnotic to accelerate and improve the recuperating of extreme injuries and reduce the excruciating pains for his patients. If somebody is seriously burnt, there will be damage to the tissue, and the body reacts with inflammation. The patients are hypnotized to forestall the soreness. His patients heal quite rapidly and with less scarring.

There are a lot more instances of how the mind can directly and physically influence the body. We realize that chronic stress can cause stomach ulcers, and a psychological shock can turn somebody's hair to grey color overnight. In any case, what I especially like about this aspect of hypnotism is that it is an archived case of how the mind positively and medically influences it. It will be somewhat of a miraculous event if the body can get into a hypnotic state that can cause significant physical changes. Hypnotic trance without anyone else has a profound physiological effect. The most immediate effect is that subjects discover it deeply relaxing. Interestingly, the most widely recognized perception that my customers report after I have seen them—regardless of what we have been dealing with—is that their loved ones tell them they look more youthful.

Cybernetic Loop

Your brain and body are in constant correspondence in a cybernetic loop: they continually influence one another. As the mind unwinds in a trance, so too does the body. When the body relaxes, it feels good, and it sends that message to the brain, which thus feels healthier and unwinds much more. This procedure decreases stress and makes more energy accessible to the immune system of the body. It is essential to take note that the remedial effects of hypnotic don't require tricks or amnesia. For example, burns patients realize they have been burnt, so they don't need to deny the glaring evidence of how burnt parts of their bodies are. He

141

essentially hypnotizes them and requests that they envision cool, comfortable sensations over the burnt area. That imaginative activity changes their body's response to the burns.

The enzymes that cause inflammation are not released, and accordingly, the burn doesn't advance to a more elevated level of damage, and there is reduced pain during the healing process.

By using hypnotic and imagery, a doctor can get his patients' bodies to do things that are totally outside their conscious control. Willpower won't make these sorts of changes, but the creative mind is more grounded than the will. By using hypnotic and imagery to talk to the conscious mind, we can have a physiological effect in as little as 20 minutes. In my work, I recently had another unique idea of how hypnotic can accelerate the body's normal healing process. I worked with a soldier in the special forces who experienced extreme skin inflammation (eczema). He revealed to me that the quickest recuperation he had ever made from an eczema episode was six days. I realized that the way toward healing is a natural sequence of events carried out by various systems within the body, so I hypnotized him and, while in a trance requested that his conscious mind follow precisely the same process that it regularly uses to heal his eczema, however, to do everything quicker.

One and a half days after, the eczema was gone. With hypnotic, we can enormously enhance the effect of the mind. When we fit your hypnotic gastric band, we use the same strategy of hypnotic correspondence to the conscious mind. We communicate to the brain with distinctive imagery. The brain alters your body's responses, changing your physical reaction to food, so your stomach is constricted, and you feel genuinely full after only a few.

What Makes the Hypnotic Work So Well?

Some people think that it's difficult to accept that trance and imagery can have such an extreme and ground-breaking effect. Some doctors were initially distrustful and admitted that his patients more likely than not had fewer burns than was written in their medical records. The cures he effected had all the earmarks of being close to marvelous. It took quite a long while, and numerous exceptional remedies before such work were generally understood and acknowledged.

Once in a while, the cynic and the patient are the same individuals. We need the results, but we battle to accept that it genuinely will work. At the conscious level, our minds are very much aware of the contrast between what we imagine and physical reality. In any case, another astounding hypnotic marvel shows that it doesn't make a difference what we accept at the conscious level since trance permits our mind to react to a reality that is independent of what we deliberately think. This phenomenon is classified as "trance logic."

Trance logic was first recognized 50 years ago by a renowned researcher of hypnotic named Dr. Martin Orne, who worked for a long time at the University of Pennsylvania. Dr. Orne directed various tests that demonstrated that in hypnotic, individuals could carry on as though two opposing facts were valid simultaneously. In one study, he hypnotized a few people so they couldn't see a seat he put directly before them. Then he requested that they walk straight ahead. The subjects all swerved around the seat.

Notwithstanding, when examined regarding the chair, they reported there was nothing there. They couldn't see the seat. Some of them even denied that they had served by any means. They accepted they were telling the truth when they said they couldn't see the seat, but at another level, their bodies realized it was there and moved to abstain from hitting it.

The test showed that hypnotic permits the mind to work simultaneously on two separate levels, accepting two isolated, opposing things. It is possible to be hypnotized and have a hypnotic gastric band fitted but then to "know" with your conscious mind that you don't have surgical scars, and you don't have a physical gastric band embedded. Trance logic implies that a part of your mind can trust one thing, and another part can accept the direct opposite, and your mind and body can continue working, accepting that two unique things are valid. So, you will be capable to consciously realize that you have not paid a huge amount of dollars for a surgical process, but then at the deepest level of unconscious command, your body accepts that you have a gastric band and will act in like manner. Subsequently, your stomach is conditioned to signal "feeling full" to your brain after only a couple of mouthfuls. So, you feel satisfied, and you get to lose more weight.

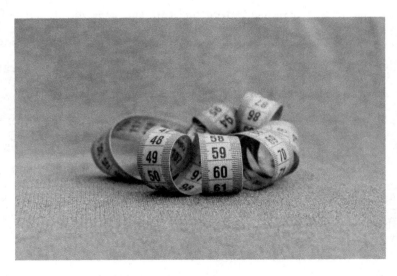

Chapter 23   Women are Different from Men

The basic principles of weight loss are the same for both genders: you burn more calories than you consume, but the factors that lead to a caloric deficit that causes weight loss are not the same. Men and women are different. They are biologically diverse and emotionally varied. These differences are significant because both biology and psychology are essential for successful weight loss.

Different Bodies

There is no need to explain the physical differences between men and women. The body composition of men and women, that is, the proportions of muscle, bone, and fat that make up the body of men and women are very different. A typical 154-pound man has 69 pounds of muscle, 23 pounds of bone, and 23 pounds of fat (the rest is organs, fluids, etc.). A typical woman weighing 125 pounds weighs 45 pounds of muscle, 15 pounds of bone, and 34 pounds of fat. Overall, men are genetically programmed to have muscular build up with heavier bones than women. Conversely, the female body is designed for higher fat content.

Technically, the meaning of overweight and obesity is based on excess body fat (Body Mass Index or BMI is used to categorize the person's weight). Again, the gender is different. Obesity in men is defined as 21-25% body fat and obesity as 25% or more. Obesity in women is defined as 31-33% body fat and obesity as 33% or more. From a biological point of view, men should be lean in appearance, and women should be fat, so men and women of the same size and weight should have very different body compositions. Given the physical differences between sexes in terms of body composition, it is not surprising that body fat recommendations differ between men and women. Men are recommended a range of 12-20% fats, and women have prescribed a range of 20-30%. Because of their different body composition, losing weight gives men a biological advantage over women.

Different Minds

Men and women don't have the same physical and psychological build-up. Differences based on emotions between men and women are an exciting area. John Gray's 1992 book "Men are from Mars, Women are from Venus" attracted people's attention and sparked a debate on the inherent differences between men and women in communication, addressing problems, and causing conflict. Psychologists are not the only ones interested in how mental processes differ between women and men. Much work is also done in the world of basic research. Every year, more and more are learned about the relationship between mental processes and physical functioning, especially concerning neurotransmitters. A 2006 article even states that men smile less than women, were due to how their brains were programmed.

It is well known that chemical behaviors in the brain influence our actions in food and physical activity. Although little is known about these signals at this time, there may be differences due to gender. The brain is associated with the potential effects of obesity and gender, so the more we learn about how the mind affects mental health, the more appropriate treatment options will be developed. The mental aspect of weight and weight loss cannot be overemphasized. The basic physiology of weight loss is relatively simple. To lose weight, you are required to drop more and ingest fewer calories. One needs to know that at the heart of permanent weight loss is the behavior of eating, exercising, and thinking. There is a clear distinction between men and women when it comes to weight loss.

Health Risk for Obese Women

Women and men share the health risks of certain diseases, but some weight-related health problems are found only in women. Weight loss seems one of the most important ways for women to overcome these problems beyond the potential health risks. Example:

Polycystic Ovary Syndrome (PCOS) is a condition that can affect a woman's fertility and is associated with obesity. Health professionals recommend weight loss as the first treatment for PCOS because studies have shown that losing weight improves productivity.

Besides, obesity is a risk factor for Gestational Diabetes. Studies show that a weight loss of just 10 pounds can significantly reduce a woman's risk of developing gestational diabetes.

Adult obesity and weight gain are also known risk factors for Postmenopausal Breast Cancer. In an analysis of a large group of women in Iowa, researchers found that weight gain at childbearing age, or preventing weight gain in overweight women combined with weight loss, was healthy during those years. It was concluded that maintaining a healthy weight reduced the risk of being diagnosed with breast cancer later.

Overweight negatively affects both genders' psychological health but appears to be more emotionally stressful for women (Emotional Stress). Studies manifest that women are less satisfied with weight and overall body shape than men. And most women's dissatisfaction with weight begins early in life and continues into adulthood. Why? At least partially, the answer lies in an attachment to the lean body for women in almost all societies.

Weight watcher researchers often hear women say they feel that others judge them by their appearance (thin and attractive), not by what they are capable of and what they can do. Where do women get this belief? Most beautiful women in magazines and big screens are extraordinarily thin people, and extraordinary thinness is a measure of beauty for many women. This seems to be primarily a woman's problem.

A study that asked men and women for their ideal body shape and asked how they thought of their bodies compared with their ideals was generally satisfied. In contrast, women consistently viewed themselves as more substantial than their ideals and expressed a desire to lose weight. Unfortunately, this very thin waif figure is unrealistic (and unhealthy!) And can't be achieved by most women. As a result, many women lose self-esteem and develop a negative body image associated with depression.

So, instead of focusing on being extremely thin, one should focus on maintaining a healthy weight. Now, we will finally move to actual weight loss techniques for losing extra fats. We will be focusing on the root of the problem, the brain.

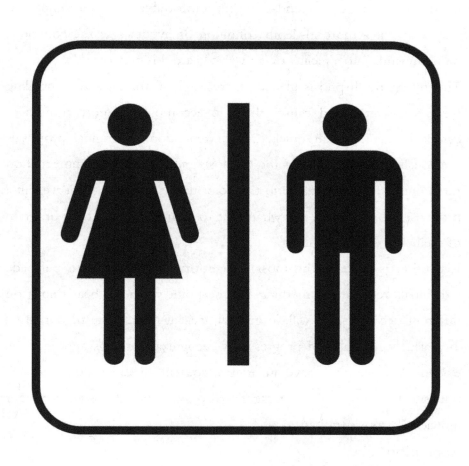

Chapter 24   The Repetition is the Secret!

The brain adores repetition since its recognizable - and natural is ameliorating. One reason repetition works are for a similar explanation - the dull hypnotic recommendation gets comfortable to the customer, and they arrive at a more in-depth condition of hypnosis as the conscious mind unwinds into a feeling of 'ah we've heard this previously.'

This makes the hypnosis meeting increasingly charming and compelling for the customer and causes them to accomplish a more prominent degree of achievement quicker. With repetition of original proposals previously, during, and after the hypnosis meeting, the recommendation turns out to be recognizable to the point that it becomes what we call a propensity for the mind - or what I like to request an executable program of the brain.

Repetition is perhaps the most straightforward approach to persuade individuals regarding something. At the point when we hear things on different occasions, we will, in general, trust it more. It turns out to be increasingly natural, and progressively recognizable things appear to be evident. Yet, we must have an original contention and realities to back our situation up, isn't that right? Also, we should have the other individual's consideration!

Repetition rule

Rule: If something happens frequently enough, I will, in the long run, be convinced.

How it functions

Play it once more, Sam. Music rehashed gets under our skin. Commercials rehashed replay themselves when we see the item. Repetition of things distinctly affects us.

Example

Our brains are great example matches and prize us for utilizing this accommodating ability. Repetition makes an example, which, therefore, and catches our eye typically from the outset and afterward makes the solace of commonality.

Recognition

Repetition makes a recognition, yet does commonality breed disdain? Even though it can occur, actually commonality prompts preferring in undeniably more cases than it does to hatred. At the point when we are in a grocery store, we are unmistakably bound to purchase natural brands, regardless of whether we have never attempted the item. Sponsors know this well indeed.

Not shortage

An impact that can happen is that repetition nullifies any shortage impact, making something at first less alluring. When I work with a well-an individual, my underlying condition overawed may before long be supplanted by the aversion of their irritating propensities. With time, in any case (if they are not very repulsive), I will presumably become acclimated to them and even get the opportunity to acknowledge and like the better pieces of their temperament.

Understanding

Repetition can likewise prompt comprehension, as it gives time for the penny to drop. What form might the outset be abnormal after rehashed presentation turns out to be clear and reasonable?

This is significant for organizations carrying inventive new items to the market where clients may look at first new to the thing or its use.

Memory

Recall learning your augmentation tables at junior school? We need to rehash things more than once for them to at last sink into our recollections. Our transient memories are famously present moment and can overlook something (like an individual's name) in under a second. Repetition is often one of the things into longer-term memory and is also an essential technique for learning.

Persuading

A few people simply need to do things a few times before they decide. Consider the last time you purchased a couple of shoes. Did you pick them at that point put them da few times before giving them a shot? Did you return to attempt them once more? Assuming this is the case, you are following after some admirable people. Numerous individuals need to rehash things a few times before they get persuaded. Multiple times is an average number.

Bothering

We can likewise get convinced in a negative redundant manner. All youngsters realize that if they rehash a solicitation frequently enough, their folks will collapse. Some recollect this when they grow up and get hitched - the annoying mate is an incredible symbol.

Daze

Repetition is additionally a reason for daze states and is like this a premise of hypnosis and hypnotic procedures.

At the point when you are figuring out how to do self-hypnosis, you'll have to utilize hypnosis contents to achieve the objectives you have set out for yourself. Through hypnosis, you will find the capacity to improve numerous parts of your life. Materials will permit you to arrive at your subconscious mind with positive affirmations and repetition.

When utilizing content for hypnosis, it's critical to use them. Negative articulations will make your mind see the exercises you are attempting to stop before viewing your messages to change. You would fortify the very propensities you are endeavoring to prevent. Instead of utilizing contrary explanations, use invigorating, positive articulations to point your subconscious the correct way.

Your contents ought to likewise be in the dynamic or current state, without reference to the past. You can't change the past; you are attempting to change what will occur later on. Abstain from utilizing action words that identify with the past tense. Keeping your announcements clear, positive, and straightforward will provide your precise subconscious orders, which it would then be able to follow.

Self-hypnosis causes you to make recommendations that will influence your subconscious mind for it to work, you should rehash your proposals to engrave these on your subconscious mind. It might likewise be useful to go astray from your set expressions once in for a little while, utilizing somewhat various words to affirm similar expectations.

A dynamic and definite methodology will help put you out and about toward your objectives. In case you're attempting to shed pounds, you may express that you are shedding pounds every day to arrive at your objective weight objective. Give yourself a timetable to work with, and show your goal plainly. If you simply represent that you will get in shape, it doesn't set a definite intention. You can customize your content by continually utilizing "I" instead of "you." This will assist with making them increasingly viable. Repeating your announcements unobtrusively using the pronoun "I" will better affect your subconscious.

Actual contents are useful to increase the comprehension of how you can give yourself proposals. Your proposals ought to be valuable for you and novel to your motivations. The contents you use will assist you with utilizing and comprehend the different ways you can speak with your subconscious mind.

Utilizing sentences of fluctuating lengths can help make your objectives understood to your subconscious mind. Longer sentences are more earnestly for your brain to see, so don't utilize excessively protracted phrases. Short and medium proclamations will shield your content from appearing to be repetitive.

Self-hypnosis can push you to reconstruct your mind successfully by quickly talking with your subconscious. Your subconscious mind puts together its musings concerning your feelings. You can change your temperament and adjust your conduct or propensities if you use contents in a positive and re-confirming way. Utilizing legitimate proclamations for your hypnosis contents is fundamental to arriving at your objective.

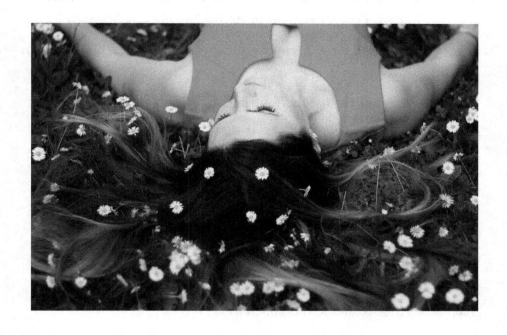

Chapter 25   Mistakes to Avoid

Mistake # 1: Deleting fun foods

"I never take cheese," " I stopped chocolate completely," "Unthinkable to have sweets at home." These little declarations of war, we have heard them all, even pronounced. However, determination is not the key to lasting weight loss.

Mind control over food is the fundamental error, arguably the heaviest and also the most common. By deciding not to eat the square of chocolate that you adore, you switch to cognitive restriction. Nutritionist. In other words, it's the start of a relentless match against your body.

And this control is fragile. A smell, tiredness, a blow of depression is enough to overcome it, sooner or later. Above all, instead of learning to recognize hunger, satiety, gustatory pleasure, you are moving away from natural sensations. We can even end up filling our hunger with a dish of green beans to succumb to prohibited food.

At the time of "cracking" (hearty dinner, snack, etc.), we enter a vicious circle:

1 / "I shouldn't, I'm going to get fat."

2 / "I will not eat more of the week."

3 / "I overeat before being deprived of it."

Not sure, moreover, that this pattern is not repeated for several days in a row. What is more, the experience of two American researchers shows that we will eventually gain weight. According to their results, after a snack (a milkshake), the people tested spontaneously adjust, without calculation, the portions of their next meal. What the "restricted eaters" are incapable of.

The solution:

No longer believe in "foods that make you fat." For this, the nutritionist recommends an exciting exercise. A person who always ends lunches and dinners with yogurt or fruit, perceived as "authorized" foods, can replace them with two squares of chocolate, the famous "prohibited" food. By keeping this rhythm for six days (weighing before and after), she will have lost weight or, in any case, will not have gained it! Because, in terms of calories, the two squares of chocolate (dark or milk) are below the intake of fruit or yogurt. Result: chocolate will no longer be a "devilish" food.

The person will even find the desire to eat fruits and dairy products because they are right and not because they "make you lose weight.

Mistake # 2: Obey the rule of three meals a day

We have been told enough to believe it: you have to eat three meals a day. Better still, a king's breakfast, a prince's lunch, and a poor man's dinner. The golden rule is much simpler and natural: you have to eat when you are hungry. We just haven't shown a relationship between the number of meals a day and weight gain.

Then, a morning calorie is the same as that of midday or evening. Studies have not shown that the body would assimilate cheese, butter, fish, fries, yogurt, fruit, protein, etc. differently depending on the time of day, which has been observed in people who practice Ramadan. "They consume the whole day's food ration all at once, even in the evening or at night. However, after a month on this diet, unless they are too rich, they do not gain weight.

The solution:

It is up to everyone to see whether they need to eat in the morning or not, a lot or a little. However, not forcing yourself to breakfast does not mean allowing yourself to throw yourself into anything at 11 am in the cafeteria or bakery. If the stomach is starving, it is better to wait until lunch while crunching an apple or taking a banana.

What your brain will deduct itself from the next meal. Be careful, however, to make the difference with snacking! We eat because we are hungry. We snack because we want to eat. But small snacks are often minimized.

Mistake # 3: "Believe" in light

Consumption of these products has only increased. Have people become less fat? No. "We now know that light and sweeteners will not solve overweight, obesity, and diabetes.

Diet products only "flatter the brain": you know you are eating a lower calorie product. But you lose in pleasure what you gain in satisfaction. A dietary cookie, "to taste, it's no longer a treat. And the 10 to 15% fewer calories compared to a normal cookie will not make a major difference, "he continues. Not to mention that, when it comes to salty snacks, "the lightened diet had the effect of distorting our taste," notes the nutritionist. Bread crumbs with fish flesh and a little oil nothing to give us spontaneously want".

The solution:

The war against sugar is no longer necessary. To his patients, Dr. Cohen advises instead to keep it, choose real sweets, and, for drinks, coffee or tea, add Stevia, a natural sweetener, for the most addicted palates with a sweet taste.

Mistake # 4: Eating too much industrial product

You apply to the letter the proportions that nutritionists recommend. But industrial or "processed" products are a real obstacle to weight loss. Breakfast cornflakes, for example, have nothing to do with grain from farmers' fields.

Children's brands have even recently been compared to junk food because of their high sugar content, a bowl may contain more than a donut, according to an independent American organization. Whatever the brand, cereal petals have a high glycemic index anyway, promoting an insulin spike and poor hunger control.

All forms of sugar that pass quickly in the blood consumed at breakfast are responsible for some vertiginous appetite before lunchtime. In this case, opt in the morning for a meal based on "rye bread with a salty touch (ham, cheese, fish)."

The solution:

Whenever possible, prefer raw foods that you prepare yourself. "Instead of a tray of ready-to-eat grated carrots, you can buy the bag of already grated carrots at the supermarket, and even the vinaigrette sold next to it. It's all about dosing yourself.

Nutritionists rely on the energy values of food alone, not those of prepared meals. When a doctor advises a yogurt at the end of the meal, it is natural, not with fruit, coulis, caramel, or other. "This type of yogurt is the equivalent of three basic yogurts, 150 calories against 50," says the research director of Weight Watchers.

Mistake # 5: Running away from the bread

Bread makes you fat? No more than the rest. Regardless of the nature of the calories, it is their excess in the quantity that causes weight gain.

Moreover, in 1900, the average consumption of bread was 900 grams per day (against 110.5 g in 2010) without the era being marked by the emergence of overweight. Depriving yourself of it does not promote weight loss. It occupies a specific volume in the food ration. And eliminating it means it's going to be replaced by other foods, probably even more energetic.

The solution:

Keep it to accompany the meal or taste, with a knob of butter (better than a cookie!). Whole or made from rye flour, it is even one of the foods to be consumed "without counting" from the Weight Watchers ProPoints2 program.

Mistake # 6: Not being followed or encouraged

This is one of the elements of the success of the Weight Watchers method: regular meetings to take stock, strengthen your determination, discuss your difficulties, share recipes, solutions, tips, then go back to " real life "and hold on.

The slimming program websites were not mistaken; all of them have a monitoring or coaching system based on e-mails, reviews to send back or explanatory videos.

This supervision of patients will soon be by text and will become daily. At mealtime, we will receive a reminder of the type: "Remember to balance your plate in three-thirds: vegetables, starches, proteins.

The solution:

The traditional consultations with a general practitioner, a nutritionist or a dietitian in flesh and blood also have their card to play. During the meeting, they will have our full attention, and then we will have less easily lied.

Mistake #7: Setting an arbitrary weight

You cannot - unfortunately - do what you want with your weight. Worse, there is no measuring instrument to determine which one it would be legitimate for everyone to claim. The only thing we know: the body will do everything to stay there! As

with hormone production or body temperature, it is an internal regulatory system.

Also, to reach or maintain a figure, not eating when hungry amounts to "fighting against inexhaustible and obstinate mechanisms. In other words, we will end up losing, inevitably. The weight of form is that which one reaches by listening to oneself. Because the very function of appetite is to "help maintain a balanced weight," says the nutritionist.

The body is exact; it calculates to the nearest calorie according to our needs and our expenses. Just as he knows precisely, once the taste detected in the mouth, the quantity of mince pie, endive salad, or salmon toast that we need. Tame your hunger, it works.

We recognize it by its particular manifestations: hollow in the stomach, gargoyle belly, nervousness, difficulty concentrating, spinning head. But the pure desire to eat, if it is upset, can cause anxiety, which signs are very close - wrongly - to those of hunger.

The solution:

Skip breakfast and postpone breakfast a little more each day to familiarize yourself with the range of sensations that range from the desire to snack until hunger. It is also she who must be in command during the meal. "We do not tighten up because we love, but because we are hungry.

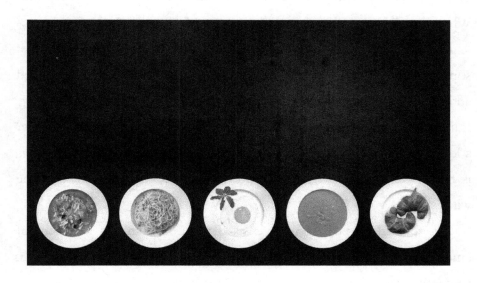

Chapter 26　Understanding Emotional Eating

Most people had eaten at one time or another for emotional reasons. When there's the tension, it can be the go-to feeling. I recall several times when one person would say to colleagues, "I'm hungry-who wants to get something with me (meaning something sweet)?" We were all exhausted and knew nothing but eating.

Eating to control emotions can end up having some negative effects over a long time. One of the main issues with using food to manage emotions is that it can lead to weight problems, and a lot more problems come with weight.

Eating for emotional purposes is used to soothe any of a variety of emotions like depression, rage, disappointment, loneliness, or boredom, to name a few. Emotional hunger isn't the same as physical hunger (the real reason for eating), and you're looking for food to meet emotional needs. We know that food cannot fulfill an emotional need, as it is intended to relieve physical hunger.

The beginning point for emotional eating is to learn if you're getting involved in it. Verily, many people are unaware of what they are doing, believing that they are overeating. The foods chosen for emotional eating tend to be the ones you would find comfort foods: high in fat, salt, and sugar. Here are some emotional eating signs:

· You eat when you're not hungry.

· Eat when you feel like you are.

· Eat-in silence.

· Eating afterward and feeling guilty.

· Overeating, and not knowing why.

· Eating to keep yourself feeling better.

· For no apparent reason, craving a snack, and feeling you can't live without it.

Emotional eating can be stimulating because, at first, it tastes good, and there are all the optimistic feelings about how much you want or need it. The good feelings (relief, calm) from emotional eating will only last for a certain amount of time (one minute to hours) followed by a turning point where you experience the following situations:

· Appointed guilty.

· Feeling humiliated.

· Feeling irritated that you are overdoing yourself.

· Feeling a revival of the initial sensation causing the binge.

· Feel angry that you've lost weight or maybe gained weight.

The result is that emotional eating doesn't relieve the primary emotion that sent you to the food. Understanding this is the starting point for this behavior to shift. Keep it for yourself. Often compliment yourself that you're "getting it" now. You can feel the need to beat yourself to do so for too long. However, this thinking cycle does not help you in any constructive way but instead brings you back to overeating because you are mad at yourself for overeating (a circular cycle).

How to Stop Emotional Eating?

Some of us have participated in emotional eating for some point or another. Emotional eating occurs if we eat to soothe wounded feelings or cope with a stressful situation. Emotional eating can occur after a hard day at work, a fight with a loved one, or when the kids run around the house crying. The first step to avoiding emotional eating is to become conscious that it is occurring. Ask yourself how you feel to stop a significant amount of tension. Recognize the symptoms of discomfort or tension. Find a way to convey the feelings efficiently so they can be published. Holding in negative or hurtful feelings may lead to a binge later on. Stopping to evaluate your emotions during the day can also help you pause before reaching for unhealthy foods.

Second, preventing causes. Think back to the last emotional eating moment. What happened just before you'd eat? Remember not being hungry and feeding anyway? Do you still eat after a difficult job meeting or dispute with a co-worker? Identifying and preventing emotional-eating activities can help deter potential occurrences.

Third, try doing something else while eating happens. By monitoring your emotional state during the day, you will be conscious of when emotional eating will occur and seeking solutions to it. When eating fattening foods makes you feel confident and relaxed, build a list of other habits contributing to the same feelings. Exercise is an important way to promote positive feelings. Other suggestions like hot baths, reading a good book or watching your favorite movie. Keep the activity list on your refrigerator to remind you of alternative ideas should a deficiency occur. Journaling is another way to avoid emotional eating.

Tracking all day long feelings, anxieties, fears, and emotions will help you recognize causes. After keeping a list for a day, look back for specific feelings that made you eat emotionally. Recurring things like job stress that require action to alleviate tension or situations that make you feel stressed. Another strategy to reduce emotional eating is to cut your portions in half. If you've had a busy day and have a meal, place half-sized portions on your plate and assess how you feel after eating. If you're still hungry, you might eat more, but if you're feeling depressed and looking for warmth, take a moment to consider your motives. Assessing your appetite and emotional state will avoid over-eating. Stop comforts like white bread and processed sugars. These foods cover negative emotions and cannot satisfy you until the meal is finished. You need to drink a lot of water during your meal. Recognize when you're complete and stop.

Finally, if you feed mentally, forgive yourself. If you keep thinking negatively about yourself, you're just accepting more tension and the opportunity to eat emotionally. Bad eating habits take years to establish and are uncorrectable overnight. Work for small goals and reward yourself when you enjoy something other than food.

Weight Loss Hypnosis and Controlling Emotional Eating Behaviors

Trauma and Stress

When a particular type of trauma or stress occurs in your life, many people become weighty. Divorce, death, and even unstable families and friends make many people feel relaxed feeding. After stress, your emotional eating patterns are in place, and your relaxation is a natural pattern for you. One of the main goals of hypnosis of weight loss is to retrain the brain to overcome these ingrained behaviors.

Emotional Hunger

This emotional appetite is not just due to stress and trauma. Emotional hunger also leads to adolescence, events that arise with peers, and learned behavior. Most overweight people eat to relieve the pain or fill a hole in life. It feels so good to eat, and sometimes you feel guided by food when everything else is out of control. Hypnosis in weight loss aims to remove these mental causes so that you do not consume foods.

True Physical Hunger

Many people have forgotten what real physical hunger is due to emotional eating habits. When you clear your mind of these negative learned habits, it is easy to know when you are hungry. It is a slow phase, and real hunger does not just strike you out of the blue. You can feel lightheaded and lethargical when your stomach sounds rumbling; this is because your brain signals that it is hungry. If you get these signals, it means that the time has come to eat and avoid starvation. However, real hunger is hard to recognize these emotional stimuli. So it is a must turn to a method that will help you quickly!

Weight Loss Hypnosis Could Be the Key

Hypnosis of weight loss is an effective treatment that can help you to eradicate mental deprivation and emotional eating patterns for right from your life. You can go beyond computational models that have held you back for many years by merely getting into a relaxed condition and listening to audio files that help you reframe your thought. Would it not be helpful to reprogram your mind and body in another way to manage stress and emotional eating? Wouldn't it feel wonderful if you could act differently seamlessly so that you can accomplish your objectives?

Beliefs and How They Effect Weight Loss

Does your conviction hold you back? There are several schools of thinking regarding a belief. But ultimately, a belief is what we really "think" or "learn." The negative side of an idea is that our life experiences shape all our values, from childhood. Some of us heard derogatory comments from those around us when we grew up, and people might have said stuff like 'you've just got big bones' or 'being in your family overweight flies.' We may have believed some of them, even without realizing it. A conviction isn't merely about 'knowing' to be true. We can 'think' and make it a belief.

The meaning of "belief" is somewhat hazy. Beliefs are learned but can be mixed with our own hands. This is one reason the word knowledge has so many schools of thought.

Applying Belief Change to Weight Loss

Having a changeable belief unlocks the possibilities to use the knowledge to lose weight. This brings up belief's 'strength' issue. If we believe enough to do something, we're motivated to do it. It doesn't matter how our views have become our values; as long as we know they're all changing. Everything our values belong to us, no-one else. It's up to us to act and change those values we're no longer comfortable.

Changing Your Belief System

If we change our system of values, we change ourselves. Believe it or not (no pun intended), once people believed the planet was flat and if you sailed too far to see you'd fall off the bottom, nowadays we'd laugh our socks off if anyone asked us. That's the funny thing about beliefs, especially old ideas, that they can harm us more than they can support us- if we let them. We will remain in our old behavior patterns because we don't think we can do anything else.

It's a self-fulfilling prophecy: if you imagine what you've always thought you're doing what you've ever done, you get what you've still got.

Ask yourself, what would you need to believe to be real to lose weight?

Since your values impact your life tremendously, but when you take steps to change them, you will make incredible improvements in your weight to life.

This is an exercise to help you change your beliefs.

1. Can you think of a belief that you know, for instance, I'm a good driver? When you can't believe in an idea, ask when you feel the day follows the night?

2. Have you got an image, a feeling, or a sound? Which qualities did you experience in the picture, feeling, or audio?

3. Think of a small conviction that you want to change 4. Take the characteristics of the belief that you know to be real and add them with the belief you want to alter.

5. Make an image of the idea that you want to change the light, big, three-dimensional, bring it right before you. Now enter the note of the image what's different?

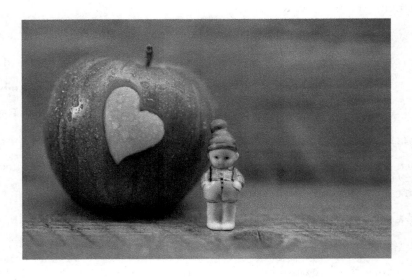

Chapter 27   Intuitive Eating

What Is Intuitive Eating?

Intuitive eating and mindful eating are frequently used replaceable, yet their functions and practices differ. Mindful eating is being aware of the whole eating experience. It requires one to focus on their food and their feelings. However, intuitive eating relies more on one's intuition. One must pay attention to the gut instinct they have. They must learn to eat for physical reasons instead of emotional reasons. This relies on one's ability to understand their internal hunger and satiety cues. Although mindfulness can assist with understanding these concepts, one must rely on intuition to feel this. Mindfulness is the process of understanding how to use these concepts. Intuitive eating is the concept itself and may be used alongside mindfulness.

Intuitive eating is not about restricting oneself to a specific diet. It's not about counting calories, weighing yourself every day, or worrying about macros. Those may contribute to overeating and emotional troubles. When doing this, one is just disconnected from themselves. They think more about numbers than how they feel. Although they may have an ideal waist size, look fit in photographs, or weigh their perfect weight, they may not be truly happy.

Intuitively eating requires the individual to pay attention to their hunger, not their boredom. It teaches people not to feel guilty about enjoying themselves and eating their favorite food. This helps to promote emotional wellness. It's important not to think about the numbers or any foods that make one feel guilty. It is more about listening to the body, which is the natural way to eat and live. It relies on internal cues as opposed to external signals. This will help the individual determine how much they should eat, what foods their body needs, and when to eat.

On the other hand, those who undergo a diet are likely to be unhappy. They will restrict themselves to eating certain foods. When this occurs, they are likely to crash at some point. While dieting, people are following what works for others' bodies. However, each individual's body differs. Everyone has various wants and needs, and those must be fulfilled differently for each person. People may eat certain foods because they're generally regarded as "good" or "healthy," but it is important to eat what makes the body feel good. One should let go of any anxiety or grief over certain foods and find out what helps to provide them with energy and happiness.

How to Eat Intuitively and Implement Intuitive Habits

To eat intuitively, one must abandon the "dieting" mentality. One must learn not to focus on weight loss or numbers in general. They must not feel guilty for their lack of progress towards losing weight. You may have books or magazines with dieting tips; get rid of them. Diets are just fads. They contribute to gaining weight more often than losing weight. Rid yourself of dieting influences. If you follow any dieting pages on social media, unfollow them. Take control of your existence instead of letting diets take control of your life. Surround yourself with positive messages regarding health and food. Cut out any negative individuals in your life that bring you down. Instead, surround yourself with positive health influences. Stop trying to chase after diets with the same results. Start fresh and reset your body and mind.

Truly listen to your body's sense of hunger. This is a naturally-occurring process that signals when it is time to eat. Eating is necessary for life. It is important to remain your energy up. You must be able to learn when your body needs to be refueled. Much like a car's gas light may go on, your body will start to send you apparent signals when it must be refueled. If you ignore this signals, your body will respond. Eventually, your body will become more desperate for food and begin craving some foods. You may also feel the need to binge or otherwise overeat to compensate for this prolonged hunger. By feeding yourself at the proper time, you are allowing your body to be adequately fueled.

Similarly, you should understand the concept of fullness. You shouldn't feel obligated to eat when you don't want to or need to. You should also not feel guilty for leaving any food uneaten. Listen to your body and understand when you are full and have had enough. It is also essential to distinguish between fullness and satisfaction. You may be comprehensive but not satisfied. Often, we will crave a particular food and still be "hungry" until we finally eat them. Instead of listening to our bodies, we will usually "feed" that craving other foods. The body, however, will still be hungry because it is not satisfied. Satisfying that craving can often prevent one from this overeating that occurs, and it will usually take less food to satisfy yourself.

You must also make peace with all the food. Eating one donut won't take you from a healthy weight to obesity. When you restrict yourself to certain foods, your body will crave the off-limits foods even more. You may feel trapped and will feel guilty about consuming any of the "taboo" foods. By disallowing oneself to have certain foods, you will feel deprived and begin developing deep cravings. When you do finally consume that food, you will likely overeat and feel guilty once more. You should not categorize foods into what is good or bad. This will only lead to guilt.

Eating should be an enjoyable experience, yet it can become an activity that causes anxiety when one labels their food or criticizes themselves.

With intuitive eating, one must also pay attention to their emotions. Emotional eating occurs as a result of these emotions. Instead of coping with emotions using food, you should find another and healthier way to handle these emotions. Although the food may help with feelings, it may not be such a great idea. Often, it won't help. It is just a temporary distraction for a bigger issue. It is also really unwise to use eating as one's primary coping mechanism. There should be different ways to help yourself feel better.

Reject vanity. With intuitive eating, one is focusing on how their body feels. If you only care about how your body looks, you may not even be truly healthy. You should not criticize your body or dislike yourself. A healthy body comes along with intuitive eating and exercise. However, one should not change their habits purely out of vanity purposes. It is essential to recognize how much it matters to treat your body well. You're only given one body in your life, so you must honor it.

The same is true for exercise. Not all of us are supposed to be (or want to be) bodybuilders. It's okay if you don't like running. You should build a fitness routine that you like. That way, you'll enjoy exercising and will even look forward to it! This means that working out will become a fun activity instead of seeming like a chore. You should also pay attention to how exercising makes you feel. This is why to do it. You will have more energy, you may sleep better, and you will have more motivation.

Intuitive eating is all about abandoning the typical ways that one loses weight. You do not have to follow a particular diet. There's no "perfect" workout routine. It's all about you. It's about what you like. It's about what makes you feel good. You must pay attention to your body and how everything you do makes you think. Although there are certain foods out there that are higher in nutritional value, you should go off of how you feel. Are the foods you eat satisfying? Are the foods you eat tasty? Of course, you may want to try putting more nutritious foods into your diet. However, you shouldn't do so because you feel obligated to or because you would feel guilty otherwise. It should be because you want to. It should be because you feel good after eating them. You must also recognize that your diet as a whole is what matters. Over time, your diet should make you feel good. It isn't all or nothing. Having some French fries or soda here and there is okay. Allow yourself to love what you eat and not feel so guilty about what you eat.

Intuitive Eating Effects

Intuitive eating has several positive effects on the body. It will lead to higher self-esteem and better body image. This is because instead of being fixated on your weight, waist size, or the foods that you eat, you will pay attention to how you feel. You will feel good and therefore know that you're treating your body well. You will feel much better about yourself after intuitive eating than you could ever think with any diet or exercise routine. You'll follow the right path for your body, not how someone else created for themselves.

You will feel more satisfied with life. In general, you'll learn how to pay attention more to what you want in life. In addition to your physical health, you will know what makes you happy and what doesn't. It will help you to feel much better about your life. The idea of not feeling guilty for doing what others are doing will genuinely help you be more satisfied with your life. You'll stop comparing yourself to others and paying attention to numbers. Life will be more about how you feel, and if you're happy, not what others think it should be.

You will become more optimistic. In addition to feeling more satisfied with life, you will feel happier overall because you are doing what you like. You won't pay attention to negativity. Surround yourself with those people who are also positive and optimistic. Life will be more about enjoying yourself instead of following someone else's blueprint. You will view life as something that you are excited about, not something you should be better.

Intuitive eating will significantly help your mental health. You will become better at coping and will develop better coping mechanisms for your emotions. This will also lead to a lower rate of emotional eating.

Those who implement intuitive eating also see physical results. Lower body mass indexes have been found with those who eat intuitively. It works! The right body will come with emotional eating. Those who eat intuitively also notice higher HDL cholesterol levels and lower triglyceride levels. Those who eat intuitively will also decrease their amount of cravings and reduce the likelihood of overeating. Because one will learn how to fill and satisfy their body, they won't feel the need to compensate by bingeing or by overeating in any way, giving in to cravings.

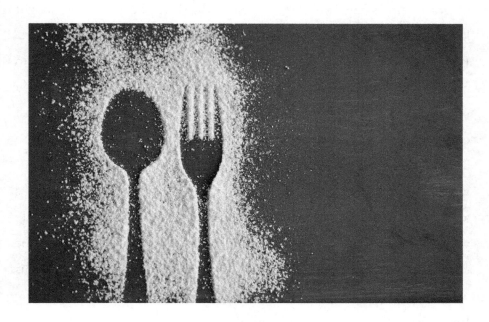

Chapter 28 Motivational Affirmation

Motivational affirmations are phrases, sentences, or even words that will enable you to stay positive, be focused, and highly motivated. You need to choose these affirmations and use them on your daily basis. They are of great help as they will help you to meditate correctly on your weight loss. You can only reduce weight when you stay focused and positive. Being true to yourself and getting motivated every time will enable you to control your weight. Even though these affirmations are numerous, you need to take a look at the ones I have detailed or illustrated the most common ones in the below paragraphs. It is good to note that, these affirmations, you can use them each morning after just waking up. They will sincerely help you to jump-start your day in a much higher note. It is a challenge thrown at you that you better try this and see how your life will drastically change. Your mindset will shift, and you will only be thinking positively. You will only be staying focused on your life, and this will increase your esteem within and outside your external world.

Below are the examples that you need to go through with much keen.

You must embrace success. In every kind of situation or no matter the condition you are facing with, tell yourself about success. You need to talk about being successful every morning. The word "you can't" should not appear in your mind. Everyone has excuses. Some excuses emerge from fear of not trying. You need to stay focus and embrace the successful part of you. Don't get overwhelmed and overtaken by negative thinking about your success story. I challenge you to recite this affirmation every time you wake up. You will realize how important it is not only to your body but also in your external world. You need to feel unstoppable and fail to look at your excuses for not being successful. Negativity here is a BIG NO for you.

You must always be calm when faced with conflict. Conflicts are issues that always take you back to where you were. Conflict will automatically kill your daily morale leading to weak contributions of your abilities, especially within the organization and other sectors of life. You should try as quickly as possible to brush off annoyances easily. You must always agree with all sorts of disagreements so that the argument can end there. Tell yourself that you are more significant than you are facing, and this should not drain you physically. Staying focused with a fit body and soul will make you lead a positive life.

At last, your weight will be highly controlled. You need to have that habit of doing this any time you are facing any conflict. It will only help you to stay positive and highly productive under your capacity. Reciting this affirmation every morning will be of great help. Try it as many as possible and help yourself to stay calm, relaxed, and comfortable.

You must choose to show love and gratitude every day. You need to know that life is always short, and concentrating on negativity is not good. It won't go well with you. It will only derail your success. After all these, you must radiate elements of joy to yourself and have that love of your body. Showing all kinds of gratitude will enable you to lead a happy life. It will affect not only you but also the people around you. You must embrace this no matter what happens. Staying scorned and having negative thoughts only ages you as quickly as possible and leaves you with a body shape you never wanted. Be happy always, and show love to the surrounding. You must try this and believe me, and you will have a change within the next few weeks.

You must be impressive to others. Staying positive in life is an excellent deal to yourself. Use anything under your disposal to impress those who are around you. You need to be positive in everything to be as positive as you can and never underrate yourself. No one sent a letter to be born in a certain way, so you need to accept yourself the way you are. It will enable you to stay focus and lead a real-life every day. You need to develop this habit of saying this affirmation to yourself as it is of great help. It will also help you to start your day with big morale and a notch higher.

You are free to develop your reality. Realities are things that are with us no matter what happens. Therefore, you must strive hard to create your reality. No one is supposed to create you one since you are in a better position with much knowledge about yourself. You must have a choice and choose wisely in every kind of situation you might get yourself herein. Remember, nothing should stand in between you and your happiness peak. That apex of goodness should be your cup of joy, and no one should prevent you from creating this form of reality to you. Choosing your reality every day will make you stay positive and entirely focused on life. Besides, it will be of great help as far as your body is concerned. Remember to note that your life ultimately depends on the realities within you. You can lie to people around you, but believe me, and you cannot lie to yourself. Therefore, it will be of great advice that you keep this affirmation as it will help you live and stay positive. In the end, this will automatically reflect on your body shape and image.

You need to shed off any unimportant attachment. Unimportant attachments are things that no longer have any effect on your life. These are things that will only let you down, thus derailing your life goals of achieving a mind-set full of happiness. Your future success depends heavily on this, and for you to get at that position, you will need to detach yourself from anything that might let you down. You must note that anything might also mean any person. We have people in our lives that always try very hard to put us down. These types of people are afraid of your success in life. They will try their best to pull you down, no matter how hard you try to embrace only positivity in your life. It is time to get yourself going and void them like the plague. Remember, you must live and not only live but choose a pleasant experience. It will only be possible if you manage to refuse anything or anyone that is holding you back. Since I have said this, it is now my wish that you may practice this affirmation and use it as your routine daily. Practice makes perfect, and you will only realize that when you train.

You are enough just as you are. You must release that demonic notion of having comparisons between you and others. For you to stay specific, you must have some success standards. After developing all these, set your own goals and ambitions. Your vision should relate to your mission in life. After all these, you can now judge yourself using the basis of your success. Those rules and regulations you created in your success standards should enable you to judge yourself accordingly. Just know you are just enough the way you were born. You are a complete soul, and no part of you is lacking. So never try to make a comparison with others. You should note that affirmation helps in the realization of worthiness. Within a short period, you will be able to control your body image. It will also be a great deal as it helps you achieve some of the personal goals in life, and having a sound body is one of them.

You must be in a position to fulfill your purpose. The world should know your existence, and you must be ready to show your achievement.

Showing your accomplished goals will need some positive deeds that lead to a successful life. On most occasions, people who trend are our trendsetters. They trend because of having done something positive or negative. They are then known all over the world. However, in this motivational affirmation, you need to focus on positive things. You need to be a trendsetter in showing the whole world what you are capable of offering. If you have been employed somewhere to sweep, you must clean until the country president cuts his journey to congratulate you. Achieving your best is always one decisive way to succeed and lead a happy life free from stress and distress. Remember, this affirmation reminds you that no one has that power to stop you from doing or rather fulfilling your purpose in life. Sharing this thought every morning when you wake up will eventually get you somewhere. You must now stay focus and have this habit of telling yourself that no one can prevent you from achieving.

You must be results-oriented. In your daily life, you need to stay focus in life. Your primary focus should be on your results.

To achieve this, you must be able to create some space for success. Get more success in your life. Avoid any derailing excuses that will only demean your reputation, thus lowering your success rate. Offer yourself these phrases every morning, and you will be in great joy for the rest of the day. You need not hold on excuses for failing to achieve something. Be yourself and have the ability to struggle until you reach that success in life. It is through this that your mind will have settled, giving you peace of mind. Peace of mind will enable you to lead a stress-free experience. It will reflect in your body image.

Be control of your won happiness. Happiness is a characteristic of life that will initiate your feelings and moods towards a positive experience. It is like a gear geared towards your prosperous life. Staying positive here will be of great importance, and for you to realize this, you must take control of your happiness. Responsibility is a virtue, and being responsible will make you bold enough to face all kinds of situations. Your joy is your key to success, and no one should tamper with it. Make happiness your priority and be responsible for it. You must let no one make you angry. Angriness will only induce you with emotional feelings that will eventually affect your life more so your body image. Having seen this, you must now be in an excellent position to embrace this affirmation. Take it as an opener to your morning and employ it entirely in your life.

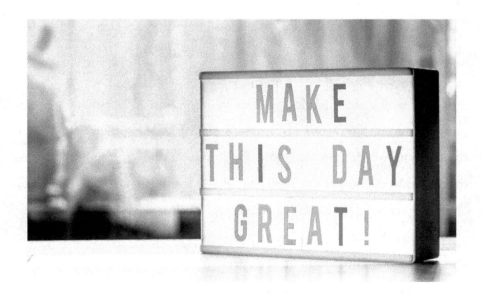

Chapter 29 Sleeping better: Making your Body Light

In every one of the Hypno Slim sessions, I additionally utilize a ground-breaking sleep-inducing process that I have by and by created and called Creating Your Light Body. This procedure urges you to relinquish all your undesirable considerations, pictures, pictures, and profound cell recollections to identify with your weight and identify with nourishment. In mending these pictures, I utilize the representation of light to assist you with making another light body; a body that capacities in flawless agreement, so your digestion and each cell inside your bodywork immaculate well-being. The more significant part of your Hypno Slim sessions will be incorporated in any event called Creating Your Light Body. This procedure is also rehashed twice for the most extreme impact.

The Ultimate Hypno Slim Program incorporates eight Hypnosis chronicles, in addition to intuitive warm-up works out.

1. Intuitive Warm-up Exercises

These activities are intended to heat your subliminal personality before you start tuning in to your Hypno Slim session. Your subliminal nature is that ground-breaking some portion of your mind that we will access during your hypnotherapy sessions; this is the piece of your brain that envisions, that fantasies and that enables you to make ground-breaking, constructive and lasting changes to how you think, feel and act. Changes that will push you to all the more effectively and that's only the tip of the iceberg make your optimal immaculate body easy.

2. Unadulterated Motivation

The most significant piece of any effective, enduring change is an inspiration. At the point when we hear "change," our mind opposes typically – it's a piece of our body science and not something we can without much of a stretch warms up. That being stated, this hypnotherapy session will revamp your body's intuitive response to change. Lastly, bond all the fundamental strides to make you wake up and state, "this is the day I venture out arriving at my weight reduction objectives!"

3. Passionate Eating

For a considerable lot of us managing weight issues, bogus hunger is a huge issue. It's simple for thin individuals to state "simply don't eat!" yet when your body's getting every one of these signs about how invigorated and fulfilled it will feel after drinking that sugar-loaded, charged bubbly drink, or by eating that euphorically liberal chocolate bar – it's tough NOT to give feelings a chance to disrupt everything!

This session will focus on wiping out those bogus food cravings and educating your body on the best way to eat how you were destined to – eating when you're eager and eating for sustenance. How much better do you feel when you've completed that chocolate bar or a pack of chips? This is the ideal opportunity you will discharge all the old psychological weight that has made you clutch your abundance weight. Over and over, I have seen incredible and positive changes happen due to this session. I would need to state this is one of the most dominant sessions of the whole program.

4. Gastric Band

This session offers a progressive new thought in the entrancing clinical field. Similarly, like a gastric band, the medical procedure takes out an abundance of weight through substantial alteration – gastric band hypnotherapy works at the intuitive level to assist you with thinning down step by step, aside from without the cost, recuperation, and symptoms.

Gastric band trance has been demonstrated to create the equivalent and once in a while preferred results over gastric band medical procedure – without the medical process. It may appear to be trying to accept, yet this shows precisely how incredible trance can be with changing conduct and shedding pounds. In this mesmerizing, I utilize explicit systems to retrain your cerebrum in ways that leave it persuaded you have experienced specific medical procedures and that you have a real gastric band setup. The consequence of this hypnotherapy approach mirrors the aftereffect of the medical procedure. You feel full more rapidly, which encourages you to abstain from indulging.

5. Altering the Band

Likewise, with its carefully embedded partner, a hypnotherapy-based gastric band additionally should be balanced. Fortunately, it won't require a touch of cutting, testing, or join and, once more, is altogether done in the brain. I'll tell your psyche precisely the best way to imagine the band altering. Your weight keeps changing, and your frame of mind toward nourishment movements to a reliable equalization of control and sustenance.

Let my words manage your psyche into a profound, loosened state, so all recommendations are met with zero opposition, and the gastric band can work freely to assist you with getting more fit easily.

6. Good dieting

Longings are your body's method for attempting to get something it most likely shouldn't have (like refined carbs, salt, synthetic substances, handled nourishment, etc.). It's so used to getting what it needs, at whatever point it needs that, similar to a grumpy baby, it will attempt to pitch a fit. It does this not by shouting and beating on the floor but by flooding your brain with pictures, scents, tastes, and a persistent want to make you yield.

Be that as it may, with this hypnotherapy session, you'll not exclusively have the option to step your longings into the ground, yet besides supplant those yearnings with reliable other options. You may not feel that grapes could fill in for chips – however, with the privilege of guided words and feelings saturating your psyche, they will.

7. Exercise Motivator

Indeed I'm going to state it; the feared 'E' word. A significant piece of any effective get-healthy plan includes venturing up your degree of physical movement.

Let's be honest. When you return home in the wake of a monotonous day of work, cooking a feast, encouraging the family, tidying up and preparing for the following day – the exact opposite thing you need to do is work out.

With the intensity of hypnotherapy, you can build your craving and assurance to practice every day. In this session, you will figure out how to appreciate the expanded vitality that originates from each endorphin moving through your body each time you work. Envision how refreshing you will feel when you step up every morning with the longing to move your body in some reliable manner. When in any event, hearing, thinking, or seeing the word practice propels you to your very center.

8. Reward SESSION Think Yourself Thin

The more you envision yourself as the slim individual you want to be, the more rapidly this will end up being your world. In this free mesmerizing chronicle, you will utilize the intensity of your intuitive personality to wash away indeed your abundance fat and make your optimal flawless body.

9. Reward SESSION Boost Your Metabolism

Your ground-breaking intuitive personality controls your body's oblivious procedures, such as managing your pulse and breathing rate. In this free trance recording, you will go into your brain's control room to enhance your digestion and assume back responsibility for your body.

Here are some great/life viable instances of Hypnotherapy related by some trance inducer for weight control:

Mary came to me since she needed to get more fit, besides, since she was feeling so wild that she wasn't getting a charge out of any piece of her life any longer. She was scrutinizing the legitimacy of her reality - the monotonous routine of getting down to business at an occupation where she wasn't valued, where she endeavored to profit, in an association with her significant other that was great however not extraordinary and had been attempting to shed more than 100 pounds for the majority of her grown-up life, at any rate, 30 years. Mary was an ordinary customer in that she had a go at everything alone to shed pounds that she could think about that appeared to be sensitive to her. There is unquestionably no deficiency of weight reduction plans and projects to be on, and she had attempted every one of them.

She realized how to shed pounds. She'd done it a lot of times previously. Be that as it may, she generally recovered it. What's more, she was burnt out on intuition about it to such an extent. She was baffled about attempting to "fathom" this issue and investing such a large amount of her energy committed to this one part of her life that appeared to have been as long as she can remember center. Mary is excellent at her particular employment and knows how to issue settle. She's fruitful in basically every other part of her life, yet this a specific something, losing the weight, just evaded her. It generally had. Furthermore, she was so baffled and tired that she didn't have the foggiest idea, whether it was worth any event or attempting any longer.

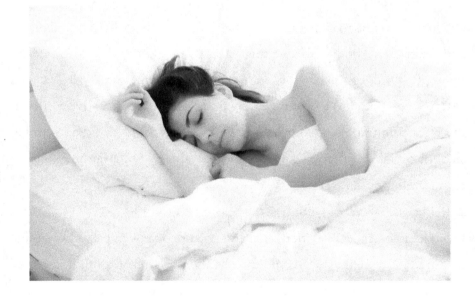

Chapter 30   Benefits of Having a Healthy Body

It is important to keep a healthy body to achieve a healthy life. A healthy body enables one to lead an active and more productive life, which directly translates to great achievements and also age gracefully. To keep the body healthy, one must have a healthy diet, subject himself/herself to regular exercises, maintain a stress-free mind, have a quality sleep, and lead a healthy lifestyle. The following are ten important reasons for maintaining a healthy body.

1. Boosts the immune system

A healthy body means that all the body processes are working at their best, and therefore all required antibodies for fighting illness are produced in enough amounts. This way, the body can fight off illnesses and protect the body from getting sick. Even though the body cannot fight off all illness, a healthy body is likely to fight off most seasonal illnesses compared to the non-healthy body. However, it is advised that if the body's immune system goes down, it is essential to avoid consuming alcohol or taking in food and drinks that are sugary. Microbes have a high affinity for sugar.

2. Reduces chances of getting any type of cancer

From a biological explanation, cancer is the uncontrolled cell division due to a mutation of the DNA within cells. DNA is responsible for giving cells instruction on when to divide, how much cells to divide, and repairing cells that need fixing. When the DNA mutates, the cells divide uncontrollably and not perform the required tasks leading to cancer. Causes of DNA mutations are either inherited genetically, biologically predisposed through chemicals causing cancer or unhealthy lifestyles like poor diet, smoking, consumption of loads amounts of alcohol, and obesity. Unhealthy lifestyles are the number one cause of cancer. A healthy body contains a normal DNA, which means a controlled cell division and also, proper repair of cells.

3. Increases the body energy level

A healthy body has high levels of energy, resulting from the work put in to achieve it. Being healthy means having a healthy diet. A healthy diet means that the body is supplied with the required vitamins, carbohydrates, and proteins. Exercising makes the body adapt to harsh treatment, and in return, every exercise session leaves the body even stronger than it was before. Enough sleep clears the mind and also gets rid of fatigue. This compilation ultimately translates to the body having high energy levels and more productive.

4. Reduces chances of being infertile

Being overweight or underweight can increase one chance of being infertile. The abuse of recreational drugs and smoking can also contribute significantly to infertility. Being overweight, smoking, and consuming loads of alcohol in men reduce the sperm count leading to infertility. Both being underweight and overweight in women also contributes to infertility. All the above-stated problems are a result of an unhealthy body. Therefore, eating healthy to avoid underweight, exercising to curb obesity and overweight cases, and leading a healthy lifestyle and minting a healthy body can go a long way in the cure for infertility.

5. Prevents stroke and heart-related problems

Stroke is where the brain is deprived of oxygen for a while, causing death to its cells. Deprivation of oxygen may be caused by blockage of arteries or rupturing of arteries leading to leakage of oxygenated blood responsible for keeping cells up and running. Among the causes of blocked arteries is the deposition of fat, blocking the proper flow of blood to the brain. Other causes may include unhealthy lifestyles and stress. Heart problems include heart attack and coronary artery disease. Similarly, coronary artery disease is caused by too much cholesterol blocking the supply of blood to the body. A heart attack is a coronary artery resulting from the heart pumping blood at a higher rhythmic pressure than the normal one. This creates pressure on the highway, causing them to rapture. The best treatment approved by doctors for both diseases is exercising, leading a healthy lifestyle, having enough rest, avoiding stress, and also adopting a healthy diet. Doctors stress keeping our bodies healthy as we can fight off illnesses like heart problems and stroke, among others.

6. Enhances some career choices

Careers like athletics require athletes to maintain good living standards and impressive body physique. Athletes are required to adopt a strict diet, exercise regularly, subject their bodies to enough sleep, and avoid consuming recreational drugs and too much alcohol if not a small amount. In the entertainment industry also, models and dancers are mostly required to adhere to similar living standards. These healthy standards ensure their bodies are at optimum health, and they can remain top of their careers.

7. Improves longevity

Study within time has shown that having a healthy body ensures one to achieve long life. Exercising for 20 minutes a day reduced the chances of one suffering a premature death. Healthy adjustments like proper diet are also essential to attain a long life. Even at an older age, the healthy body also means that one can carry out tasks that would have been hard if they were unhealthy or dead. It also means that one can enjoy more time with family. Grandparents get a chance to see and bond with their grandchildren because of maintaining their bodies at healthy levels

8. Helps control body weight

A healthy body is a state acquired after proper care of the body and exercises. Even without trying to lose weight, healthy living standards will ultimately lead to healthy body weight. A weekly schedule of a few hours of exercise and eating right will go a long way in maintaining healthy body weight. The body will have a strong immune system, prevent heart diseases, and spike the body's energy level as a result of a healthy body

9. Improves moods and feelings

A study has proven that exercising our body leaves our bodies relaxed and happy also. This is a result of the release of brain cell chemicals called endorphins. Exercising also ensures that one achieves an athletic physique, which means that one will have improved physical appearance, leading to improved self-confidence. We live in a world full of regrets and tragedies. It is essential to keep out bodies at most health for improved emotional balance and also maximum cognitive functions

10. Helps manage diabetes

There is 2 main kind of diabetes, one is where the body itself attacks the body insulin-producing cells, and one has to live on insulin shots all his/ her life and type two diabetes where the body is unable to absorb the sugar in the blood and convert it into energy for the cells. Type one diabetes is a result of poor health living standards, lack of exercise, and having a poor diet. A right diet and exercise can control the early stages of diabetes like Prediabetes and also gestational diabetes. Maintaining a healthy body will mean that the body will be able to control body insulin balance and reduce fatalities caused by Diabetes like blood pressure, heart attack, kidney failure and hardening of blood vessels

11. Improves the brains memory

A healthy body constitutes a healthy diet; a healthy diet comprises of all the food nutrients. Among these nutrients are vitamins. Vitamins, preferably C, E, D, Omega 3, fatty acids, and flavonoids, are essential in developing a brain with a good memory. A healthy diet also helps fight off dementia and decline of cognitive functions. Dementia is the loss of memory, effects on the ability to speak, think, or even solve a problem. Eating healthy will help reduce dementia that which is not caused by physical injury on the brain.

12. Strengthens both the bones and the teeth.

Maintaining a healthy body helps improve the strength of teeth and bones. It is advisable to consume dairy products for calcium three portions a day. One is also required to subject the body to physical exercises, and the most preferred one is lifting weights. A proper diet is essential, as well. One is required to consume meals rich in calcium and magnesium for healthier teeth and bones. Many kinds of cereal contain calcium while magnesium is abundantly found in legumes, nuts, whole grains and seeds

13. Boosts self-esteem

Among reasons for having low self-esteem is having an unhealthy body. We live in a world of diversity and one that is rich in different tastes in fashion. Often everyone wants to look good, but sometimes our bodies often fail us, which can be bad for our self-esteem. However, this can be changed, and our esteem boosted within no time. A proper diet would be a good start accompanied by regular body exercises and maintaining a healthy mind through rest and controlling what we think. Results take time, but eventually, one achieves a healthy body. This is more like killing two birds with one stone as one can boost their self-confidence by enhancing appearances and also obtain a state of a healthy body through having a healthy body.

14. A Healthy body improves better sleep

Often people with unhealthy bodies go through a lot of difficulties when sleeping. They often sweat a lot in cases of obesity and even find difficulties breathing when asleep. Healthy people sleep well and encounter no problems breathing when sleeping. Subjecting the body to exercises ensures the body process work right, and it burns off excess fats causing sweating during the night. Eating right and avoiding abuse of drugs and alcohol also helps achieve a healthy body. A healthy body, in turn, leads to sound sleep

15. Improves sex life in couples.

Sex is a physical act; therefore, both partners are required to be physically fit to have a good time. More often than not, once one of the partners gains an unreasonable amount of weight or both partners, they start experiencing bedroom problems. Sex is a significant aspect of all couples, and if issues arise in this area, the likelihood of separation is high. It is therefore advised of couples that they maintain healthy bodies to avoid bedroom problems.

16. Improves chances of surviving disasters and violence

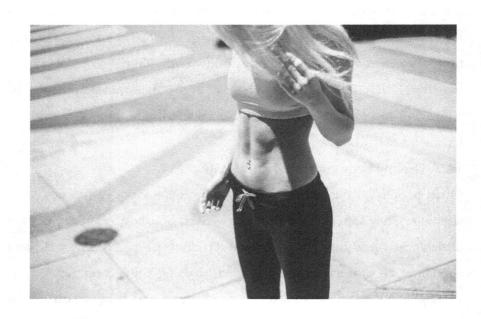

Chapter 31   Self-Confidence and Self-Love

Self-love is probably the best thing you can accomplish for yourself. Being fascinated with yourself furnishes you with fearlessness, self-esteem, and it will, by and substantial, help you feel progressively positive. You may likewise see that it is simpler for you to experience passionate feelings once you have learned how to cherish yourself first.

Self-Confidence

Self-confidence is just the demonstration of putting a standard in oneself. Self-confidence as a person's trust in their very own capacities, limits, and decisions, or conviction that the individual in question can effectively confront everyday difficulties and requests. Believing in yourself is one of the most significant ethics to develop to make your mind powerful. Fearlessness likewise realizes more bliss. Regularly, when you are sure about your capacities, you are more joyful because of your triumphs. When you are resting comfortably thinking about your abilities, the more stimulated and inspired you are to make a move and accomplish your objectives.

Meditation for Self-Confidence

Sit comfortably and close your eyes. Count from 1 to 5, concentrating on your breath as you breathe as it were of quiet and unwinding through your nose and breathe out totally through your mouth.

Experience yourself as progressively loose and quiet, prepared to extend your experience of certainty and prosperity right now.

Proceeding to concentrate on your breath, breathing one might say of quiet, unwinding, and breathing out totally.

If you see any strain or snugness in your body, inhale into that piece of your body, and as you breathe out, experience yourself as progressively loose, quieter.

On the off chance that contemplations enter your psyche, notice them, and as you breathe out to let them go, proceeding to concentrate on your breath, taking in a more profound feeling of quiet and unwinding and breathing out totally.

Keep on concentrating on our breath as you enable yourself to completely loosen up your psyche and body, feeling a feeling of certainty and reestablishment filling your being.

Experience yourself as loose, alert, and sure, entirely upheld by the seat underneath you. Permitting peace, satisfaction, and certainty to full your being at this present minute as you currently open yourself to extending your experience of peace and happiness. As you experience yourself as completely present at this time, gradually and smoothly enable your eyes to open, feeling wide conscious, alert, better than anyone might have expected – completely present at this very moment.

Self-Love

Self-love is not just a condition of feeling better. It is a condition of gratefulness for oneself that develops from activities that help our physical, mental, and profound development. Self-love is dynamic; it promotes through activities that encourage us. When we act in manners that grow self-love in us, we start to acknowledge much better our shortcomings just as our strengths. Self-love is imperative to living great.

There is such a significant quantity of methods for rehearsing self-love; it might be by taking a short outing, gifting yourself, beginning a diary, or anything that may come as "riches" for you.

Meditation for Self-Love

To start with, make yourself comfortable. Lie on your back with a support under your knees and a collapsed cover behind your head, or sit comfortably, maybe on a reinforce or a couple collapsed covers. For extra help, do not hesitate to sit against a divider or in a seat.

If you are resting, feel the association between the back of your body and the tangle. On the chance that you are situated, protract up through your spine, widen through your collarbones, and let your hands lay on your thighs.

When you are settled, close your eyes or mollify your look and tune into your breath. Notice your breath without attempting to transform it. What's more, see additionally on the off chance that you feel tense or loose, without trying to change that either.

Breathe in through your nose and afterward breathe out through your mouth. Keep on taking deep, full breaths in through your nose and out through your mouth. As you inhale, become mindful of the condition of your body and the nature of your brain. Where is your body holding pressure? Do you feel shut off or shut down inwardly? Where is your mind? Is your brain calm or loaded up with fretfulness, antagonism, and uncertainty?

Give your breath a chance to turn out to be progressively smooth and easy and start to take in and out through your nose. Feel the progression of air moving into your lungs and after that pull out into the world. With each breathes out, envision, you are discharging any negative considerations that might wait in your brain.

Keep on concentrating on your breath. On each breath in, think, "I am commendable," and on each breathe out, "I am sufficient." Let each breath in attract self-esteem, and each breathes out discharge what is never again serving you. Take a couple of minutes to inhale and discuss this mantra inside. Notice how you feel as you express these words to yourself.

On the chance that your mind meanders anytime, realize that it is all right. It is the idea of the brain to meander. Necessarily take your consideration back to the breath. Notice how your musings travel in complete disorder, regardless of whether positive or negative and enable them to pass on by like mists gliding in the sky.

Presently imagine yourself remaining before a mirror, and investigate your very own eyes. What do you see? Agony and pity? Love and delight? Lack of bias?

Despite what shows up in the meditation, let yourself know: "I adore you," "You are lovely," and "You are deserving of bliss." Know that what you find in the mirror might be not the same as what you see whenever you look.

Envision since you could inhale into your heart and imagine love spilling out of your hands and into your heart.

Allow this to love warm and saturate you from your heart focus, filling the remainder of your body.

Feel a feeling of solace and quiet going up through your chest into your neck and head, out into your shoulders, arms, and hands, and afterward down into your ribs, tummy, pelvis, legs, and feet.

Enable a vibe of warmth to fill you from head to toe. Inhale here and realize that affection is continuously accessible for you when you need it.

When you are prepared, take a couple of all the more deep, careful breaths and, after that, delicately open your eyes. Sit for a couple of minutes to recognize the one of a kind encounter you had during this meditation.

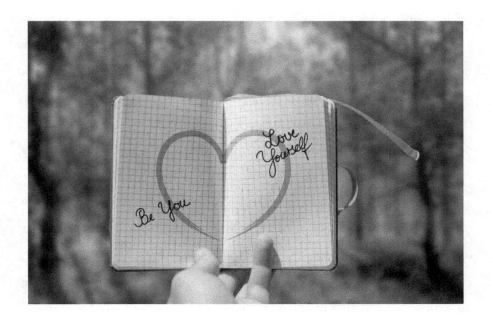

Conclusion

Hypnosis is often used for many different reasons today, something that once was thought of as a magic trick or something that doesn't work. However, looking at results curated by clients over the years, especially with weight loss, one can see that it is indeed something that can help you to get ahead in life. Apart from losing weight, it can help you overcome your fears, stress, anxiety, depression, and even support your mental well-being when faced with addiction, sleep deprivation, challenges, and more.

It also contributes as a significant factor supporting health and wellness, allowing you to practice mindfulness, which many individuals don't know how to do. It aids as a psychological treatment that can help you experience far more benefits to serve your well-being than you ever thought. It allows you to experience changes in your thoughts, behaviors, perceptions, and sensations and can be performed in either a clinical setting or the comfort of your own home.

Hypnosis has successfully proven to improve deep sleep in individuals by up to 80%, allowing one to wake up more energized and refreshed each day.

After experiencing this audiobook, you are undoubtedly aware of the incredible benefits that hypnosis for weight loss holds in store for you.

To refresh your mind about the benefits you could experience by following one of our hypnosis for weight loss sessions, our listed wellness benefits include:

• It helps to rectify sleep patterns, such as insomnia, sleepwalking, and having general trouble sleeping. If you suffer from these issues, you can learn how to relax your brain and form better sleeping patterns by following a daily hypnotherapy program. Given that hypnotherapy aids in fixing any problems related to improper sleep, it also serves your weight loss journey, as rest is required to maintain a proper-functioning body and mind. It also assists your metabolism is operating correctly, which helps you lose weight, restores the cells in your body, and ensures the proper harmonious functioning of your entire body.

• It helps to reduce anxiety and depression. Since anxiety and depression are experienced due to an imbalance of emotions and being overly affected by the daily stresses of life, hypnotherapy works by relaxing the mind, allowing patients to become in town with themselves and attain a sense of control and mindfulness in their lives. Hypnotherapy is tailored to enable you to let go of any negative thoughts, habits, and daily experiences you may have, shifting your focus on positive things. Given that many health issues stem from anxiety, including irregular breathing, high blood pressure, heart diseases, and the potential to create an overall imbalance in the body, hypnotherapy serves as the perfect option to control any stress or anxiety you may experience. As stress and anxiety are the most significant contributors to overeating, lack of portion control, and emotional eating, it's yet another reason why it can aid in significant weight loss. Since hypnotherapy is focused on fixing the mind, everything else usually aligns perfectly.

• It helps to l the symptoms associated with irritable bowel syndrome symptoms (IBS). Hypnotherapy can ultimately relieve symptoms related to IBS, including constipation, bloating, and diarrhea. It can also improve bowel movements and support a balanced metabolism, which prevents secondary disruptive symptoms, like fatigue, nausea, backache, and urinary tract issues.

- It helps you to quit addictions. Since most people turn toward addiction to help get rid of their problems as a result of stress, anxiety, depression or emotional issues, it's simple to understand why hypnotherapy can help one quit bad habits, including smoking, alcoholism, an addiction to medication or pain killers, and most relevantly, an addiction to food. Hypnotherapy allows you to train your mind to take whatever your addiction is and form a type of resistance toward it in your subconscious, which eventually translates into your conscious thinking.

- It helps to reduce chronic pain and symptoms associated with feeling unwell. Hypnotherapy's purpose is to help you overcome many obstacles in your life and make you feel like you are on the tops of the world. It serves as an excellent method to help you overcome symptoms associated with illness or stress in your body and can take your overall wellness to a whole new level.

Taking chemotherapy for cancer patients as an example, even though patients often want to give up, they shouldn't. Since the mind can determine whether we are sick or not, hypnotherapy can alter the perception and make one believe that they are getting healthier. With this positive incentive in mind, patients will only focus on getting better and not on the severity of their diagnosis. Hypnotherapy can indeed help cancer patients stay positive, and thus speed up their recovery, serving even an even higher purpose as those who lack positivity during chemotherapy are more likely to give up early and pass.

- It can help you lose weight!

After reviewing the endless benefits hypnotherapy presents you with, we can conclude that it is indeed a practice of divine intention and medicine, blissfully combined to create the best version of yourself than you ever thought was possible. Whether you're suffering from obesity, you're a little overweight; you suffer from health issues contributing to your struggle in not losing weight.

There is always a reason why you can turn you can't into a can.

In truth, losing weight is not rocket science. It is quite simple and can be achieved, no matter where you're in your life or how difficult you may think you have it. Focusing on weight loss, we have also established the importance of focusing on your overall recovery, which serves you every day.

It demands respect and will serve you even better if you can manage to resist the temptations life throws at you ever so often, and in some cases, every day. Learning principles in nutrition, such as the fact that sugar is a killer and that white-based flour carbohydrates are not your friend, can serve as a massive asset in your journey toward achieving wellness, among many other things.

To make your journey more comfortable, it's also a better idea to focus on wellness than a number on the scale. Weight loss will occur if your intentions are set right. You know who you are as a person, and so, you can either remain the same or choose to grow. Your mind is connected to your body, and the two require each other to survive, you must ensure that both operate harmoniously. Only then will you see results, survive this incredible journey, and attain success in all you wish to achieve.

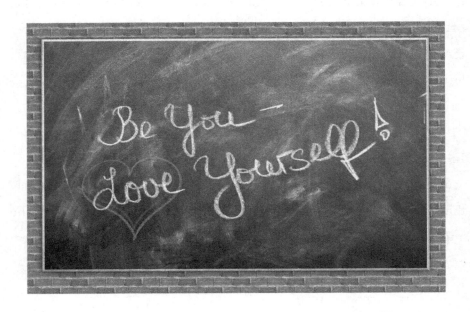